HEALTHY⁴

A Surgeon's Guide
to Health and Wellness

Thomas F Moyad MD, MPH

While the healthy4 program was designed by a medical doctor, we realize that everybody is different. We highly recommend that before implementing any new dietary or exercise routines you consult your own doctor, especially for those with disabilities or illnesses.

INTRODUCTION

The key to unlocking your full wellness potential lies within this program and within yourself.

Have you ever wondered why so many weight loss programs fail to produce enduring results? The reason is simple: Most nutrition and diet books focus on only one aspect of our health. These programs often promote losing weight by limiting the types of foods we eat or by limiting certain carbohydrates and fats. While this certainly is a very necessary aspect of dieting, it is just part of the overall picture.

Likewise, why do so many of us make a resolution to become physically fit, yet have problems maintaining a consistent exercise routine? The answer is the same. Most fitness programs focus on a single aspect of our health, rather than using a truly integrated, holistic approach.

Lastly, why have so many people attempted to manage their stress level or sought the aid of a self help guide, only to become discouraged by the lack of enduring results? I think you may have guessed my answer already. It's because these methods are often used in isolation. Sooner or later it becomes too difficult, if not impossible, to overcome poor habits that weaken our resolve and lead to poor health.

In order for us to achieve long-lasting health, we must incorporate four key components that make up our overall well-being. Without an intimate knowledge of these four factors, our efforts to improve our health will be limited at best.

Take diet plans, for instance. Many times they are doomed to fail right from the start. If we do not search for the root cause of overeating we will have great difficulty modifying this behavior. Calorie restriction used in isolation will work for only so long before we break down and lose our mental stamina. Eventually we return to a maladaptive pattern of eating that for many is the result of unresolved anxiety or stress. Thus, we must first understand the cues to our hunger and address potential unhealthy eating habits before we can jump into a diet program.

Exercise programs are also frequently neglected or fail because they are performed in isolation without regard to proper nutrition or without considering other barriers that impede our resolve to exercise. For example, overeating can lead to fatigue and lethargy that inhibits one's ability to exercise. On the other hand, we need to obtain an appropriate amount of vitamins, minerals and calories to optimize our energy levels which will, in turn, facilitate our physical fitness routine. Another barrier to exercise comes in the form of mental or physical stress. This often leads to apathy or fatigue and limits one's ability to remain committed to a long term exercise program. However, if you learn how to manage your stress effectively, your capacity to exercise will increase substantially, as will your overall health.

Some of you may be wondering what makes the Healthy 4 program different from all the other so called "holistic" health books available today. It is important for you to understand that this book contains fundamental principles accepted by medical doctors and health professionals all across the world. The science of each of these fundamental principles cannot be disputed. However, the true power of this program comes from the integration of all the key health components. The Healthy 4 core principles have been arranged into a logical, easy-to-follow regimen designed to take each of you through a step-wise progression towards your ultimate goal of wellness. This holistic program allows you to maintain your motivation and optimize health. It does so by building a solid foundation that begins in the first chapter and is continually reinforced throughout each section of the book, culminating in a well-designed, integrative program by the last chapter. The concepts contained within this wellness program are not complex. Still, it has taken me many years to acquire the knowledge and experience used to create it. I promise, then, that as I pass my knowledge to you, you should begin to see results that will lead you to a healthier and more fulfilled life.

———

I first began cultivating an interest in holistic medicine and prevention of disease almost two decades ago, during my graduate studies in Public Health at the University of Michigan. During my training, I often questioned what we as medical professionals could do to improve health outcomes and reduce the burden of disease in our patients.

Later on, during my surgical residency and fellowship, I had the opportunity to work at the University of Michigan Hospital and Harvard Medical Center, both very prestigious surgical training programs. I learned a great deal about my profession and I was privileged to train with some of the best surgeons in the country. Although I was fascinated with the human body and surgery, my interest in promoting holistic health increased, especially when I realized that a large percentage of patients could have prevented many of their health problems if only they had the proper education, motivation and training.

Unfortunately, one significant barrier to providing holistic health in our modern medical care system has to do with the way that doctors and other health care providers are reimbursed and valued for their expertise. To say it another way, our current health care system does not financially reward or support health care providers who truly practice holistic health. Although this may seem unfair or unjust, it is the reality of westernized medicine. Rather than treating the whole patient, our current system encourages isolated treatment without abolishing the root cause of preventable diseases.

Don't misunderstand; I do believe that miracles are performed every day by those who work tirelessly within our current health care system. Our medical resources and advanced technology is second to none within western medicine. Nevertheless, the fact remains that over half of all human diseases that lead to enormous suffering and despair are totally preventable. The power to optimize your health and ultimately obtain a heightened sense of well-being is truly within your reach. By utilizing the techniques outlined within the Healthy 4 program, you can and will become healthier and happier!

As a licensed Medical Doctor and Board Certified Orthopaedic Surgeon, I still do enjoy treating diseases and acute problems requiring immediate attention. However, what I am most passionate about is helping my patients avoid modern medical services in the first place. In other words, what is most important to me is improving the health and wellness that is within all of us. The key to unlocking your full wellness potential lies within this program and, if you choose to seek it out, you will find that the key is also within yourself.

As I have alluded to, the idea of holistic health is certainly not a new concept and it has commanded much interest over the last several decades. Still, many people who genuinely wish to prevent disease and improve their health actually lack the basic resources and necessary knowledge required to do so. The health and wellness industry is as much to blame for this as any one individual.

For instance, many so called holistic health companies are focused on selling products and services rather than providing practical methods to improve wellness. The problem is widespread and can be seen in strip malls across the country, infomercials on television, and scattered over the internet. The nutritional supplement market, for example, is a billion dollar industry. We often see companies advertise their products as "holistic" or "all natural" but in no way resemble whole foods. Many of them have no proven benefit or, worse, may actually be dangerous. Even common vitamins such as Vitamin D or Vitamin E taken incorrectly or in excess can lead to harmful toxicity. So what is the consumer to do? With all the confusion out there, it's no wonder people have a hard time trusting what works.

That is not to say that all nutritional products are bad. I, too, am a believer in nutritional supplementation when used properly. In fact, I have been using certain vitamins and nutrient supplements for many years and routinely recommend a variety of them to my patients. My issue is with the industry's failure to provide a practical, results-oriented approach in today's health product market. We have neglected common sense in our quest for immediate results. I can promise all of you that a pill, powder or any other single agent will not make you a healthier person. True, some of these supplements are important nutritional adjuncts that promote health when used in combination with a viable health program. However, taken in isolation they do not work. Thus, we need to view the big picture. What we need is a good plan!

As mentioned, people often encounter mixed messages from the numerous holistic health books and guides available today. Many health companies mistakenly focus on marketing a specific type of product such as a nutritional supplement or type of exercise equipment. On the other hand, there are other programs that target only a small population of people rather than reaching out to the average person. Examples of these can be found in various hospital-based wellness programs and health insurance plans.

In fact, many "wellness" companies are created by non health professionals or, worse, professionals who aim for profit potential rather than human potential. Fortunately, as a physician and creator of the Healthy 4 program, I have been able to bridge the gap between the complementary or alternative health market and allopathic medicine. We at Healthy 4 are passionately dedicated to substantially improving the lives of our clients. We provide a unique and yet practical approach to our holistic health program that works and is readily accessible to people from all walks of life. This consistent, well-developed program is available to all people, not just a select few from a certain region or socioeconomic background. Most of the tools presented throughout this book can be used by persons from different backgrounds, regardless of age, life experiences, physical limitations or financial resources.

I have used the same fundamental guidelines and recommendations contained within this book on thousands of individuals and I have seen many success stories. The common theme that I hear over and over again from others who have followed these principles is that they feel stronger, more energetic and have a heightened sense of peace and well-being.

Of course, achieving your optimal health is not always easy and it will take dedication and commitment. One of the main goals is to transform your body and mind so that the Healthy 4 program becomes part of your daily routine. This transition period will take some time and patience, so don't expect to feel different right away. Most of you will find that, over the long run, you will begin to approach your health routine with anticipation and vigor as it becomes a natural part of your life.

The *principle components that affect our health* can be broken down into *four basic categories:*

1) **Diet**
2) **Exercise**
3) **Stress**
4) **Spirituality (Sense of Purpose)**

By the end of this book you will be able to fully understand how each of these four areas interacts with one another to either strengthen or diminish your overall health. You will begin to take control of your own health and happiness by adhering to the methods outlined in the upcoming chapters. It is vital to your future success that you realize that these four components are not mutually exclusive.

Rather, these four areas are interwoven with one another, each having either a positive or negative influence upon the other. Learning to integrate all of these components together will strengthen your resolve and increase your health exponentially.

Perhaps the best way to grasp this relationship is thru the following schematic diagram:

INTERRELATIONSHIP BETWEEN THE 4 HEALTH COMPONENTS

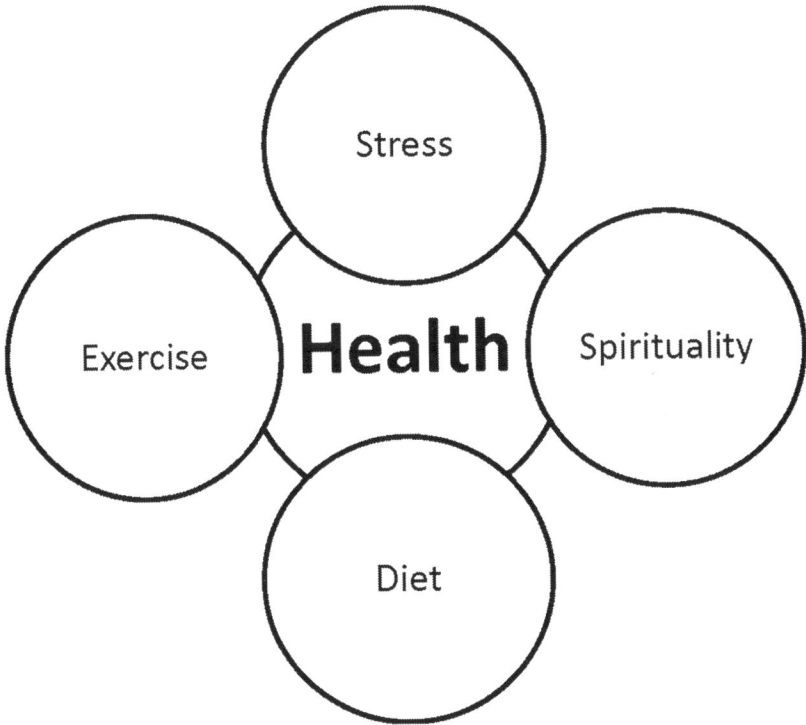

Stress

Exercise

Health

Spirituality

Diet

Some of you might be thinking that it is better to just address one problem, especially considering time constraints that we all face in our lives. Or, you may feel that it's easier — and therefore more beneficial — to focus on just one thing at a time. Some of us are inclined to believe that we only need to work on our weakest areas, as the other components seem to be "good enough." There are several reasons why these arguments do not work.

First, this system was designed to work efficiently only when the four components are integrated. It was not designed for single-component use and therefore its efficiency will be greatly diminished if not used as intended. In addition, only a simple positive additive effect is anticipated if performing an individual health component in isolation. In contrast, these four principles, when incorporated together, have an exponentially beneficial effect upon your health.

You should also realize that we all have room to improve, no matter what our level of experience. So, if you feel that you are strong in one area – for example, if you exercise daily – you will find that this program will increase the effectiveness of your routine. Additionally, by combining all four principle aspects of wellness, you will heighten your ability to maintain your routine over time and optimize your health, since consistency and longevity are the keys to optimum results.

―――――

As you will soon learn, the Healthy 4 approach to wellness is designed with the intent of providing maximum results and enduring health. Integrating proper diet and exercise, along with stress management and sense of purpose is necessary for optimal health and it serves as the backbone of this program.

By the end of this book, you will have all the necessary tools to significantly improve your health, happiness and longevity. We will examine each of the components of the Healthy 4 system and discover methods of improving these areas throughout our journey together. Importantly, we will integrate diet, exercise, stress reduction and spirituality into one comprehensive plan that is easy for you to follow. Along the way, you will be provided with many suggestions and techniques that will assist you with this program.

I strongly believe in what I call the "why first, what then" philosophy. This means that, rather than begin by telling you what you must do, my first objective is to offer valuable insight and knowledge concerning why you should take action. I want you to understand the basic concepts and relevant issues first, before using the practical tips and pearls of the program. In this way, you will believe in the program for yourself, not because I (or anyone else) have told you to do it.

As a Medical Doctor, I have always strived to use this same approach with all of my patients. I realize that people have the best chance of success when they understand the decision making process and the reason behind action. This is because clarity is a prerequisite to passion, and passion in turn leads to action. When combined with the proper plan, we are destined to succeed. Knowledge really is power!

Part of this process is to avoid a challenging review of topics intended for health care professionals. For you, the reader, this means an action plan that is understandable and ultimately leads to self improvement without all the research details and discussions. This book focuses on key concepts and practical techniques that cover the major components of health. Thus, it combines interesting facts and information along with practical applications that assist you in minimizing inefficient health practices while maximizing your well-being.

Throughout this book, we will be building a program together. At the end of the book, you are provided with a program summary which reviews all the important concepts, tips and techniques that you will learn during your journey. Never try to use this summary without reading the full content of the book first! Remember, this summary review is meant to be an outline and thus serves as a useful refresher. However, you must read the entire book to appreciate the key concepts and understand how to use this summary.

––––––

We will begin the Healthy 4 program with the diet component. In this section we will discuss monitoring and controlling your normal calorie consumption, which is the foundation of any diet and weight loss plan. "Diet" in this case is used in its traditional sense and refers to healthy eating and not a temporary program intended for quick weight loss. And, by "weight loss," we mean a permanent shedding of excess weight that naturally occurs with a healthy lifestyle.

To reach this long-term health, we will teach you how to examine nutritional labels, ensuring proper nutrition and healthier consumption. You will also learn key techniques to promote healthier eating habits. Incorporating these healthy dietary habits will assist you in maintaining your ideal body weight and provide you with the necessary energy to exercise and combat stress.

Next, in the chapters on exercise, we will put together an exercise regimen that works for you. You will learn about common barriers to exercise and how to avoid these pitfalls. You will also start to incorporate diet and exercise together to optimize your efficiency and strengthen your resolve. Some of you may consider yourselves advanced athletes, while others may be coping with certain physical limitations or disabilities. Whatever your level, there is an exercise regimen right for you. For those who have a routine, we will explore ways to modify your regimen in order to optimize your health.

Later on, we will present methods to cope with stress and you will learn simple, effective techniques to reduce the types of stress which can lead to physical and mental illness. Specifically, you will learn that not all stress is bad. We teach you how to identify potentially harmful stress and how to eliminate it from your life. The techniques and tips contained within these chapters are an invaluable part of the Healthy 4 program. Since stress reduction is an essential part of your overall health routine, we will cover common causes of stress in detail. We will then lay out a plan that will allow you to eliminate or significantly reduce the main causes of stress from your life.

In our last section, we will explore spirituality. Often seen as separate from the body, our spiritual quest is more often ignored in wellness programs. Through the Healthy 4 program, we will discover that in fact spirituality is a key component in the quest to improve our overall health and happiness. You will begin to understand that developing your spirituality, or a sense of purpose, is the glue which binds all the health and wellness elements together into a cohesive program. Along the way, we will see how these four components are interwoven and you will learn how to tie them together in order to create a healthier and more joyful lifestyle.

We are now ready to begin exploring the means to optimize your health. Our goal is to create a healthier and more fulfilling life through focused learning and participation in a truly holistic wellness program. I hope that this journey is as rewarding and enlightening for you as it has been for me and for thousands of others who have gone before you. I know that if you keep an open mind and remain dedicated to the principles outlined within this book, you will ultimately become healthier and happier. Remember, there is truly no greater gift in life than your health and well-being. It is a gift to yourself and to those who love you. You deserve it and so do they. So, what are you waiting for? Let's get started...

TABLE OF CONTENTS:

COMPONENT ONE:
DIET

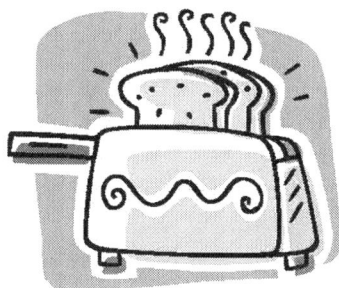

CHAPTER ONE:
MONITORING CALORIES

There are thousands of dieting books and programs on the market and it may seem extremely difficult to choose which one, if any, is right for you. Since you have opened this book, I assume you are looking for a program that is simple, practical and provides long-term results. The key to any long term results is consistency, consistency, consistency. Yes, it is that important!

One question that always comes up is, does dieting work? Of course, the answer depends on your consistency or ability to "stick to it." So, really, the question is "Will I be able to sustain or maintain this or that diet?"

Let's assume that a certain diet requires you to consume diet bars or shakes from a specific company to reduce your caloric intake. Will these foods leave you satisfied? In truth, they probably will at first because you will be motivated. But how long will this program be sustainable? For most of us the answer is, not very long at all. Quick weight loss foods are very rarely sustainable, mostly because they leave you hungry, but also because they lack all the basic nutrients that a proper diet requires. That is why many diets end up with the dieter splurging or gaining all the weight back in a short amount of time.

So, really, any diet that will be maintained is one that meets basic requirements of proper nutrition as well as provides you with the tools necessary to sustain your diet.

Let's start with the most basic principal:

THE AMOUNT CONSUMED SHOULD EQUAL THE AMOUNT USED

Human beings need a specific amount of calories per day to sustain our important bodily functions and physiologic processes. Anything more than this specific amount is wasted or stored in the form of fat. We all know how excess calories can contribute to an enlarging waistline or belly. Worst of all, it can contribute to the buildup of plaque in our arteries, which is a cause of heart disease and stroke.

Every person is somewhat different in their daily energy (calorie) requirements. The exact amount of calories that we need to maintain our body weight depends on many factors such as our lean body mass, basal metabolic rate, activity level and age. Fortunately for us, we don't need to know this exact amount. A rough estimate of our daily caloric needs is enough. Once we have a ball-park figure of how much we should be eating per day, we can modify our intake over the weeks and months.

At this point, I am giving you permission to avoid the scale. You will actually be able to visually monitor your progress throughout this process and avoid the hang-up of a particular number. As you will learn later on, there are two simple methods of self monitoring. One involves numbers (such as BMI, which we discuss later) and the other is visual. At different times, each will serve a purpose and we will eventually use both to monitor your progress.

For example, let's assume that you need somewhere around 2,000 total calories per day to meet your daily nutritional needs. This is a pretty good starting point, since the RDA (Recommended Dietary Allowance published by the United States Department of Agriculture) was based on a diet of 2,000 calories per day for the average adult. Again, keep in mind that we do not have to be exact in the amount of calories you need per day, we just need a rough estimate. Obviously, if you're pregnant or if you are an elite athlete, this may not be enough calories. For the majority of us, however, 2000 calories a day is a reasonable starting point. You can find your recommended daily nutritional requirements by visiting Nutrition.gov and searching under "Reference Dietary Intakes."

After establishing our recommended caloric intake, the next question might be "what types of foods should I be eating?" Unfortunately, the typical western diet often contains too many fats and simple carbohydrates and not enough fruit, vegetables or grains. The recommended number of these and other relevant information can be found on the USDA website and studying the revised food pyramid at www:

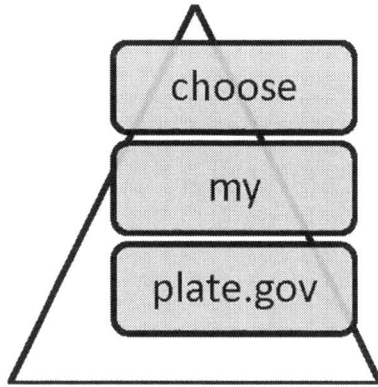

Whether you're a proponent of the older food pyramid or the newer "choose my plate" model, there are similarities between the two. In general, both of these concepts attempt to convey the message that our diet should be made up of differing proportions of food groups in order to obtain an adequate balance. Fats, oils and sweets should obviously be consumed the least. Next would be foods such as milk, yogurt, eggs, meat and poultry. The largest share of our calories should come from sources like vegetables, fruits, cereals and rice.

Later in this book we will discuss these things in greater detail, including portion sizes. At some point it is definitely worth a deeper look. For the moment, however, we are going to put off other nutritional information and concentrate on this one simple tenet:

THE AMOUNT CONSUMED MUST EQUAL THE AMOUNT USED

Once we fully appreciate this basic physiologic law, we improve our ability to maintain our body weight. Simply put, if we consume more than we need, we add to our body weight. Conversely, if we take in less than we need, we lose body weight. This may seem to be an oversimplification but it is such a critical point to maintaining proper weight that it must be burned into our memory. Once you truly understand this principle *and practice it every day*, you will begin to discover that dieting is not as hard as it seems. It will still require discipline, but the frustration and complexities that thwart so many diets will fall away.

The next step in constructing a plan requires a little math and a log book. Once you have acquired a note book to record your daily intake of calories, you are on your way to dieting and weight loss. To begin, you need to *record everything you eat, every day, for the next 15 days.* It is important for the record to indicate how many calories you consume per meal or snack, too. Now, at first glance this may sound like a lot of work, but it really is not. It only takes a few minutes per day and the information gained is absolutely invaluable.

There are some diet programs on the market that try to do this work for you by telling you exactly what type of foods to eat and how much of it you can eat per day. I believe this is where many of us go wrong. Foremost, if you are eating foods that you do not enjoy, you will not be able to continue your diet very long. If you are disciplined, you may be able to do this for a month or two, but sooner or later you will want to eat things that you do enjoy. Our goal is not to build a diet around what other people tell us to eat, but rather what we would like to consume (within reason, of course!)

Second, we cannot start by making drastic changes in our diet. First we must determine what we are doing wrong and where we stand. We cannot do this without making note of our present consumption patterns. So, for the first two weeks, you should continue to eat whatever you normally eat and focus only on how much you consume rather than alter the type of food you eat. One of the reasons for this has to do with my earlier point of *consistency*. By allowing yourself to consume foods you are accustomed to during the early diet plan, you will be able to concentrate on the program's most critical aspects. Thus, your chance of consistency and longevity will increase.

Eventually we will learn to modify our diet by eating healthier foods since there are obviously downsides to eating unhealthy foods. For instance, if you normally eat high fat, high caloric foods (i.e. cheeseburgers), you will often be hungry throughout the day because these calories add up quickly. After just a few cheeseburgers, you will have very little room to spare before your daily calorie limits are exceeded.

Furthermore, this unbalanced approach can cause a vitamin and mineral deficiency. Thus learning to balance your diet can actually decrease your periods of hunger, yet it still allows you to consume certain foods that you are accustomed to, albeit usually in smaller portions.

If you are a finicky eater, don't fret. We all have the ability to acquire a "taste" for most foods, even for the ones we may not have previously enjoyed. However, this adaptation does take time to develop and it should not be the principle focus during our initial phase of the diet plan. As the program develops, we will recommend and incorporate healthier foods, but for now, eat the foods you like.

Now that you understand the basic logic, let's return to formulating a plan. Again, for the first 15 days of this diet, eat exactly what you normally eat *without* restriction. Do not alter your eating habits or reduce your calories during this period. All you have to do, then, for the first 15 days, is record how many calories you normally consume.

Most of this calorie information is found on the food labels of the groceries that we purchase. If you often eat at restaurants, some of this information is already contained in the menu. If not, ask the wait staff or manager if they carry nutritional information on the foods that they serve. The internet also provides good information on unpackaged foods such as meats, produce and legumes.

This early objective is to assess how much energy (calories) you typically consume each day. Although it's not vital to account for every last calorie, the more information that is recorded, the better off you will be when it comes time to put this information to good use.

For restaurants that don't publish calorie information, you will have to take your best guess. This will be more challenging at first, but over time it actually becomes much easier. How does it become easier you may ask? By reviewing the calorie content of the basic food groups and ingredients, you will learn to estimate combined foods and more complex meals. This skill does take some time to develop, but when it does, you will gain a much greater appreciation and deeper understanding regarding the foods that you allow into your body.

To illustrate my point further, we will review the following example from a typical food diary:

Let's say for breakfast you have:

1 bowl of cereal
1 banana
2 slices of toast with strawberry jam, and
1 cup of orange juice

Your log book entry for that morning may look something like this:

Date: xx/xx/xx
Meal 1: 730 calories

How did I arrive at this information? Actually, it was very simple. As I said, all the caloric information on foods we buy from the grocery store can be found in the nutritional label on the package. I estimated that:

One serving size of cereal with 2% milk =	250 calories
One banana =	90 calories
Two pieces of toast with jam =	280 calories
One cup of orange juice =	110 calories
Total breakfast calories =	730 calories

Let's look at another example; this time, a snack before dinner:

One apple =	90 calories

During dinner you consumed:

Two slices of frozen cheese pizza =	280 calories
One 12 ounce soft drink =	140 calories
One cup of ice cream=	340 calories
Evening total	850 calories

Again, you will find all this information on the back of the food nutrition labels and on various online sources, including the FDA.gov site. So remember do not discard these labels if they are on the outside of the packaging until you have had a chance to write down what you have consumed.

To make your log book entries even easier and less time consuming, you may want to write only the number of total calories that you consumed for that particular snack or meal. In other words, you can simply add up what you have consumed for each meal or snack and record the amount next to the meal.

For example:

Breakfast:	400 calories
Snack:	150 calories
Lunch:	600 calories
Snack:	100 calories
Dinner:	800 calories
Daily total:	2,050 calories

In this example, you only have a few lines to record in your book every day. Again, what's most important during the first 15 days is to get an idea of how many calories you normally eat rather than modifying the actual diet, which comes later. How detailed you make your individual log book is up to you. This will depend on how interested you are in recording the information. The most important part of this step is to obtain a fairly accurate assessment of your total calorie consumption, regardless of how you record the information. Although the more detailed your log book the better since it will provide you information later on about the types of foods you are normally consuming and in what quantities.

Now, some of you may be tempted to cheat or skip ahead and avoid the process of writing down your calorie intake during the first 15 days. **DON'T.** If I have not convinced you of this already, let me say it again: This is an important step! Each step builds on the progress of the previous step, so cutting corners now means less progress in the future. Besides, what do you have to lose? It only takes a few minutes a day and minimal effort. In return, it serves as the foundation of your evolving diet. It fact, there are several critical reasons why you should perform this exercise.

First, recording your calories will allow you to get a better handle on whether you are truly consuming too much food and by how much. For some, you may need to only reduce your intake slightly or increase your activity to a modest degree. For others, you may find that you are consuming thousands of excess calories per day. Remember the old saying: Knowledge is power. Whatever your situation, this first step gives you the necessary knowledge and understanding that will be needed to modify your diet and improve your health.

In addition, you will find that with a little practice, you will be able to add your calorie intake up very quickly. In fact, don't be surprised if you're soon able to remember the energy content of many foods and drinks that you consume daily without ever looking at the labels. As I alluded to already, you can also use this knowledge when dining out, even when eating at restaurants that do not provide caloric information on their menus. This skill takes a little practice, so be patient.

Most importantly, developing a habit of studying what we eat and drink improves our awareness of what we put into our bodies, and makes it easier to modify our diet in the future. Remember, you should not expect or anticipate this modification to take place immediately. It requires both time and effort.

Finally, from a purely practical standpoint, it's easier to lose weight or change your body's shape when monitoring your calories.

Let's revisit our golden rule:

THE AMOUNT CONSUMED MUST EQUAL THE AMOUNT USED

This rule is important when trying to maintain your ideal body weight. Therefore, if you want to lose weight or decrease body fat, you may need to consume several hundred calories fewer per day than what you normally require. Over time, you will be able to see with your own eyes how effectively this works. It may take weeks or months, but it will work. Of course, if you have any serious medical problems or nutritional concerns such as diabetes, eating disorders or pregnancy, talk to your doctor about changes in your caloric intake.

As a physician with more than 15 years in the health care industry, I have seen many patients in my lifetime. The good news is that for most of you, monitoring your calories really does work if you stick to it. Of course, it is not always easy, but like many things in life that are worthwhile, it takes effort and a good plan.

Let's consider for a moment how much your car is analogous to your diet. When you drive you must fill your car with fuel (gasoline) in order for it to work. Humans also need fuel (food). How do we know when it's time to fill our cars with fuel? Well, one way would be to drive it until your car runs out of gas. Of course most of us would agree that to do this intentionally is not the brightest of ideas. (Although I must admit, I have on occasion driven "on fumes" to see how many miles I could get from a single tank!)

A much better way to assess if we need gas is by monitoring various gauges and systems, including a fuel gauge and a warning light. Similarly, we need to approach dieting through systems and gauges. We wouldn't want to wait until we pass out from hypoglycemia (low blood sugar) before we decide to fuel up. This would be like running out of gas in the middle of the road. While this isn't typical for most of us, many of us do "drive on fumes," waiting for hunger pangs to kick in before eating.

To prevent or control hunger, then, we should establish a routine pattern of consumption with fairly regular meal times. This system helps to fuel our body efficiently, rather than relying solely on hunger, which is often an imperfect gauge. Why? Because hunger involves complex thoughts and emotions in addition to basic physiologic drives. Thus, our hunger often over-estimates the amount of food we need to consume in order to remain healthy and refuel our bodies.

Taking the automobile analogy one step further, how do we know when we have enough gas to get us where we need to go? Well, we could continue to fill our tank until we see the fuel spill out from the nozzle and onto the pavement. Again, probably not a good idea if you have any environmental consciousness and are concerned with wasting money.

Instead, most of us use one of two methods. The first method is to fill the vehicle until a shut off device is activated that prevents us from spilling fuel onto the ground. This is similar to using our sense of fullness (called satiety) to decide when to stop eating. This crude method, however, often leads to problems of over consumption because satiety, like hunger, involves complex patterns of behavior in addition to normal physiologic processes in our bodies. Unfortunately, some of us don't feel full until we have gorged too much food in a very unhealthy manner, while others feel full at just the right amount. Thus, we should never rely on the sensation of "fullness" as a proper gauge. Granted, we can fuel our cars without worrying about using all the gas in the tank before refueling. Unfortunately, the human body differs from an automobile in this regard, since we can accumulate excess weight if we fuel our bodies without burning the excess energy reserves in a timely manner.

The second method one can use to determine how much fuel to buy at the pump involves estimating the total number of miles we need to drive and the approximate number of miles per gallon that our car burns. For example, if we need to drive 300 miles and we know our car can get 30 miles to a gallon, it's easy to see that we will need approximately 10 gallons of fuel. (Wouldn't be nice if every car could get that kind of mileage?) In this example, even if the fuel tank could accommodate several more gallons, we would not need to fill the entire tank since 10 gallons is all that is necessary for our destination.

Rather than relying on satiety or our sense of fullness, a much better method of monitoring our food consumption is by estimating the daily calorie requirements. This allows us to better gauge our meals and realigns our portion size with our daily energy needs. I am not saying that one must account for every last calorie that he or she consumes for the rest of their life. However, we do need to pay more attention to our calorie intake. This is why I am asking you to record what you eat and drink in your log book at the beginning of this process. With time, you will subconsciously modify your own pattern of consumption even before recording any numbers or referring to a book.

I must emphasize the importance of using this log book technique until you become intimately familiar with what you're eating and how many calories you consume per day since you will be changing the amount of energy based on trial and error. Therefore, writing this information down while you are working through the process is invaluable.

Some of you may be asking "Why is he making such a big deal about keeping track of calories? Why not just eat a sensible diet, exercise and forget about monitoring our food so closely?" The simplest answer to this question is that it just doesn't work for most of us. The main problem is in the way we have been programmed to think. That is, our idea of what is "sensible" has evolved steadily to a point where our health is now in jeopardy.

It is well known that obesity has been rising rapidly in many countries including the United States. This epidemic has become so rampant that it's even present in our young population. In fact, research now shows that obese teenagers *already* have worrisome changes in their arteries, which correlate with early signs of heart disease. It must be emphasized that these diseases are preventable. However it requires a change in the way we approach our diet and our health in particular.

It's worth mentioning again that a proper diet does involve more than just calorie counting, although it remains a big piece of the puzzle. Other considerations include the percentage of fats, carbohydrates, proteins and other nutrients in a given diet. It is also important to monitor the sodium chloride (table salt) and cholesterol content in the foods we eat. An improper balance of high saturated fats, cholesterol or salt can adversely affect our health, no matter how well we control our calories. Without a doubt, we should all strive to have a well-balanced diet to improve our health.

Nevertheless, as I have just illustrated, the major problem in most industrialized nations – including the United States – is a problem of over consumption rather than under consumption. Calorie monitoring is an excellent tool that helps us manage our weight and combat this problem.

Occasionally, you may hear about some people who have been able to consistently maintain an ideal body weight throughout their entire life without concern for what they eat or how much they consume. However, we should view this with a grain of salt, as this is rarely the case. Sometimes, and for a variety of reasons, certain individuals do not want to admit to others that they think or act in a way which is good for their own health. Certain people would like you to believe that dieting and health just come easy to them. This can be seen in some of our celebrities and in certain cosmetic advertisements for example. Mass media sometimes gives us the impression that beautiful and perfectly fit people surround us everywhere we look. The truth is that even those people who seem to have the ideal body often work very hard at obtaining those results. Furthermore, the methods that are used by some models and celebrities are far from healthy and can actually cause physical damage. The bottom line is that maintaining a healthy body and lifestyle does take effort.

For the very few individuals who truly eat poorly or consume huge amounts of food and stay trim, there may be a very good reason behind this pattern. There are some medical conditions which cause an abnormal increase in metabolic activity and make it difficult for a person to gain weight. This can occur with diseases of the thyroid gland.

It this case, we would never want to consider these individuals fortunate because of their ability to eat whatever they want. They actually may be dealing with a serious health problem. Additionally, even if a person can consume very large amounts of food and never gain weight, they still need to follow an appropriately balanced diet to ensure they ingest the proper nutrients. For example, consuming a large number of certain types of fats and avoiding important sources of fiber would be unhealthy for anyone, even for those with an ideal body weight. However, for the vast majority of us, the reality is that we must always think about the amount we eat as well as modify our practices in order to maintain a healthy weight and lifestyle.

On the opposite end of the spectrum, we often hear people complain that they have trouble with weight gain because their body does not burn as many calories as the next person or that they have a slow metabolism. Again, it's important to take everything with a grain of salt. While it is true that each person's metabolism is different, for most people the simple fact is that they lack the correct knowledge or skills to maintain a proper weight and healthy diet.

The fact that one person's metabolism may work "better" than another is truly irrelevant for most of us. Remember, our bodies are all different. The key is that our consumption must match our needs. You should expect that some people have calorie needs that far exceed yours and vice-versa. What is important is that we must all base our own diet on our individual needs, not the needs of others. If you truly understand and live by this rule, you already have won a large part of the battle.

As with all things, few exceptions exist. It is a rare individual whose metabolism is so sluggish that they need medical treatment in order to maintain their nutritional requirements or to lose weight. For most of us, even those with slower metabolisms, it is possible to maintain a healthy diet and weight without the need for medical intervention, but we must have a well-rounded plan that includes proper diet, routine exercise and the right mind set and will to execute it. This is exactly what the Healthy 4 program is all about. This book will help many people who want to lose weight, which is a significant benefit. However, the main objective of integrating proper diet, exercise, stress reduction and spirituality into our daily routine is to maximize our overall health and well-being. Thus, the essence and true benefit of this program provides us with so much more than diet or weight loss alone.

CHAPTER TWO:
FOOD LABELS AND CHARTS

In addition to a well-balanced diet, another important caveat to consider when examining food groups and their nutritional labels is the actual quantity of food in the container. In particular, the so called **serving size** is a critical concept to grasp. The serving size is the measured amount of food that is used to calculate the nutritional and calorie content of a given solid or liquid food. In other words, the number of calories and the percentage of fats, sugars, proteins, minerals and vitamins that are listed are all based on this designated serving size. For example, one serving of breakfast cereal is often listed as one cup of cereal. Do not assume that one serving of a particular food is equal to the actual serving that you consume! This is a common mistake, since people often tend to *under*estimate how much food they consume.

When monitoring your calories, especially during the first few weeks and months, you need to be as accurate as possible when evaluating your food. Simple foods will be easier to assess while more complicated meals will be more challenging. For instance, if the serving size is based on a single slice of bread or single piece of cheese, this should be a piece of cake (pun intended!)

In other cases, the portion size is based on a table spoon or cup which can be harder to quantify. In these cases, you should use these actual measuring tools. You may be quite surprised by just how inaccurate your estimation of a tablespoon or cup can be, especially early on in the diet program. It is not uncommon to underestimate the portion size that we consume by 50 percent or more. Therefore, always try to use a measuring cup or the actual spoon size (teaspoon or tablespoon) that is used to calculate a given serving size when possible. This allows you to more precisely assess your caloric intake. As a result, the validity of your food log will improve and the estimate of your daily food consumption will be much more accurate.

I realize that you may not want to measure everything you eat or drink for the rest of your life. I am certainly not asking for a lifetime commitment. However, I am asking you to be as accurate as possible and measure your intake whenever possible during the first few months. With practice, your estimation skills will improve and you will learn to unconsciously modify your own portion size, if necessary, and become much more in tune with your body. This allows you to avoid excessive consumption and makes it easier to maintain a more optimal body weight.

Let's now examine several basic food charts with their associated caloric content. Once again, you can find all of this information by reviewing the nutritional labels printed on a given package or container of food. The following list is by no means all inclusive and other nutritional content has purposefully been omitted here to illustrate a few noteworthy points. However, these charts are very useful in the sense that it allows you to review some of the common food trends as well as the actual calorie content of a variety of foods. You can also find this information on the health resource page of our web site at www.Healthy4.com.

PROTEIN RICH FOODS	CALORIE CONTENT
6 ounce fish fillet (halibut)	165 cal
1 cup 2% milk	140 cal
1 egg (medium size)	40
4 ounce shrimp (1 & quarter cup)	80 cal
12 ounce chicken breast	360 cal
5 ounce (small size) nonfat yogurt	120 cal

CARBOHYDRATE RICH FOODS (complex carbs and simple sugars)	CALORIE CONTENT
1 cup pasta (penne)	400 cal
1 cup pasta sauce	140 cal

1 waffle (whole grain)	90 cal
1 cup frosted corn flakes	110 cal
1 slice bread (whole grain)	90 cal
1 table spoon jelly	50 cal
1 apple (medium size)	80 cal
1 cup 100% orange juice	110 cal
1 (12 ounce) can of cola	140 cal

FOODS RICH IN FAT	CALORIE CONTENT
1 slice (1 ounce) cheese	110 cal
10 inch small thin crust cheese pizza	750 cal
1 cup mint flavored ice cream	340 cal
1 chocolate chip cookie	80 cal
5 pitted black olives	45 cal
1 table spoon cream cheese	45 cal
1 table spoon lite cream cheese	35 cal
1 table spoon sour cream	30 cal
1 table spoon lite mayonnaise	50 cal
1 table spoon peanut butter	100 cal
1 table spoon vegetable oil	120 cal
1 table spoon olive oil	120 cal
1 table spoon butter	100 cal

Examining these tables closely, one is able to note several important trends and valuable insights. First, never be fooled by crafty marketing and advertising campaigns that use words like "reduced calories" and "lite" in their language. Often foods that use these labels are extremely high in fats or calories in their original form and continue to remain high in fats or calories even under their "lighter" labels.

For example, take a look in the last table, Foods Rich in Fats. Notice that one tablespoon of cream cheese is 45 calories and one tablespoon of "lite" cream cheese is 35 calories. In this case, this reduction is fairly small. What's more is that this "lite" version contains calories that are still derived mostly from fat. Next, look at the lite mayonnaise listed just underneath. One tablespoon is 50 calories. That doesn't seem to be "lite" to me either. The point here is that you should review everything you eat and decide for yourself if it is good for your diet, rather than letting others influence you to buy their product with misleading or unregulated claims.

On the other hand, I am certainly not against all foods that use these persuasive descriptions. Every bit helps, really. What I am most concerned with is that this type of food marketing strategy tends to cause complacency or cause a person to overestimate how much they should consume. You must always think in terms of "apples to apples" not "apples to oranges". In other words, if you normally use one tablespoon of mayonnaise, do not use two of the reduced calorie kind.

Another important aspect of dieting is to limit the intake of high fat or high calorie condiments and spreads such as butter, mayonnaise, margarine and other dressings. Take another look at the bottom several oils and spreads in the last table, Foods Rich in Fats. Here we can see that a tablespoon of olive oil has the same amount of calories as a tablespoon of vegetable oil. Butter also contains a very high number of calories.

The point here is that oils used for cooking and dressings are all high in calorie content and all are made of 100 percent fat. While these fats have their place in our diets, we do need to be careful of the quantity used. When recording these, you will realize how quickly the calories add up. In fact, many of us could be dressing or preparing the meals we eat with hundreds or perhaps thousands of extra calories without ever realizing it.

To combat this habit, try eating your foods "naked." No, that doesn't mean that you should dine with your pants off. (You can, but it would have no bearing on caloric intake!) What I do mean is that you should try eating your toast without butter for instance. Some people refer to this as "dry" or "plain." If that bothers you try substituting the words "healthy" or "unspoiled."

What sounds more appetizing, eating something dry or eating something healthy? Hmmm...... I think I prefer the healthy food instead. How we choose to label something really does affect our perceptions and actions. But we'll examine this in much greater detail in later sections of the book. For now, just realize that having a preference for a particular food is often acquired. If you haven't tried already, start eating your foods without the dressings or oils that you may normally use. Over time, you just may develop a taste for foods without needing to cover them with unnecessary calories.

That is not to say we should never eat fats. Some claim that certain fats are good for us, such as fish oil. There are opposing views on which fats are healthy and which are bad and these arguments make it difficult to know what to consume. In truth, the answer lies somewhere in between and we will return to the discussion in greater detail in upcoming chapters.

The next interesting and significant point that we can learn from the food charts is that it's not always readily apparent how many calories are contained in a given food. Take, for instance, the calorie content of pitted black olives. Just 5 small olives contain 45 calories. These types of foods are easy to over consume since they have a high caloric content per volume of food. On the other hand, an entire head of romaine lettuce is often less than 20 calories. This is a very low calorie food compared to its volume. The take-home message is to always check the labels if you are unsure about the nutritional value of a certain food. Many times we will discover that the salt, fat, cholesterol or calorie content is much higher than we previously thought.

One of the last topics that we should discuss concerning the nutritional charts is to review our liquid intake just as thoroughly as our solid intake. By looking at the chart labeled "Foods Rich in Carbohydrates," we can see that a small can of cola or soda contains 140 calories. At first glance, this may or may not appear to be a large number. Keep in mind that liquid consumption can add up to an enormous amount of calories per day. Just 3 cans of soda or tall glasses of fruit juice per day can equal the calories of an average meal. Of course, 100% real fruit or vegetable juices are at least healthier liquids since they contain more essential nutrients and vitamins compared to a typical can of soda.

In general, however, it is best to obtain your daily minerals and vitamins from solid foods. Solids usually have a much slower transit time through your digestive tract, making you feel full longer, and taking up more space. Unlike liquids that are full of sugar or carbs, solid foods tend not to lead to hypoglycemic "crashes," either. Therefore, avoiding high calorie liquids may help reduce your calorie consumption significantly. This does not mean that you should give up drinking fluids altogether. On the contrary, adequate hydration is extremely important for your body, as it helps to rid toxins from the body and facilitate normal vital functions. Although the jury is still out regarding zero calorie diet drinks and their possible health concerns, you should consider fluids that are at least lower in calories. This is especially true if you have difficulty limiting your calorie intake to match your goals.

The safest way to reduce your daily liquid calories yet maintain adequate hydration is to drink plenty of water. Drinking water allows you to avoid the concern for harmful synthetic chemicals and does not add any additional calories or weight gain. As I have pointed our earlier, taste is often acquired and this is true for water as well as food. Because of the proliferation of flavored drinks on the market, especially so-called "energy" drinks, many people have trouble consuming unadulterated water. No worries. Eventually, you will develop a taste for water and even prefer it to many other liquids.

The final point I will make regarding these calorie charts is that they obviously do not paint the entire picture. I have said repeatedly that building a balanced diet is important and you shouldn't lose sight of this from our discussions regarding calorie counting. However, a discussion on the significant vitamins, minerals and other nutrients in food cannot be exhaustively discussed in one book. If you would like to learn more, I would encourage you to research the subject as much as you can. For the rest of us, it is enough to be aware of our basic needs and the nutritional content in the foods we eat.

Thus, it is very important to continually read the nutritional labels and record your caloric intake. As we know this is a necessary step in the diet component of the Healthy 4 program.

Why have I focused on caloric intake so much? For one simple reason: It gives the most bang for the buck! Rather than dilute your attention on an overwhelming array of facts and tasks, the intent of the program is to understand key concepts and use applied techniques in order to deliver the most concrete results and provide the greatest positive impact on your health.

CHAPTER THREE:
FATS, PROTEINS, CARBS OH MY!

In the last chapter, we briefly discussed fats in relation to overall caloric intake. Now, we will learn to understand the difference between certain types of fats and their proposed advantages and disadvantages.

DIETARY FATS:

To keep it simple, consider that all fats are made of the same two basic chemical building blocks – hydrogen and carbon. These hydrocarbons, as they are called, are bonded together like the links in a chain. Chemically the dietary fats are all closely related and their unique properties are due primarily to the way in which they are bonded or linked together.

Cholesterol on the other hand is not a fat and is chemically distinct from fats. It does, however, play an important role in the transportation of fat throughout our body. It is found in both the foods we eat (called dietary cholesterol) and manufactured in our body in a variety of forms as well. Keep in mind that not all forms of cholesterol are bad. The good type of cholesterol actually protects our heart and the bad type can damage our heart.

The two critical concepts to understand concerning the dietary fats and cholesterol are as follows: First, there are some types of fat contained in certain foods which increase our risk of serious health problems when compared to other types of fat, especially if these are consumed in large quantities. The reason that these fats are believed to be unhealthy is because they seem to have a propensity to increase the body's production of bad cholesterol. This bad cholesterol has been strongly associated with coronary artery disease and heart damage.

The second concept is that we do need a balanced diet with a certain percentage of fats, preferably more of the "good" fats. However we need to exercise some common sense. Many people in America and in other industrialized nations commonly consume too many calories in their diet, including too many fat calories. In these cases, adding more fat and calories to one's diet, even healthier fats, can be unhealthy and ultimately harmful. So the message in this case is one of moderation.

For instance, if a person consistently consumes twice the amount of food calories they require each day, this individual would miss the big picture if his or her focus was primarily on consuming "good" fats. Rather, his or her pattern of overconsumption would be the main issue and would likely pose the greater health risk.

Some of you may already be familiar with the common categories of fat: unsaturated, monounsaturated, polyunsaturated, trans and saturated fats. The last two, saturated fats and trans fats are thought to have more **adverse health effects** compared to others. Saturated fats are derived primarily from animal sources and become hard at room temperature (unlike unsaturated fats which remain in a liquid state at room temperature). Trans fats are generally man-made or altered plant-based fats, such as shortening and margarine.

Healthier alternatives include the *unsaturated, non-trans* fats such as nuts, fish oils and other sources of Omega 3 Fatty Acids (such as seeds). *Common unsaturated oils generally come from plant sources and include:*

- ➢ Olive oil
- ➢ Vegetable oil
- ➢ Canola oil
- ➢ Peanut oil
- ➢ Walnut oil
- ➢ Grape seed oil
- ➢ Sun flower oil
- ➢ Flax seed oil

- ➤ Corn oil
- ➤ Safflower oil
- ➤ Sesame oil

Less desirable fats such as the *saturated or trans fats generally come from animal sources and include:*

- o Butter
- o Margarine
- o Red meat (non-lean cuts)
- o Lard
- o Cream cheese
- o Coconut oil
- o Fried foods
- o Shortening
- o Whole fat milk
- o Whole fat cheese
- o Sour cream
- o Egg yoke

Thus, it is advisable to try to obtain the majority of your daily fat requirements from sources that contain unsaturated fats and non-trans fats. Remember, this does not mean you should consume these fats at will or without regard to your calorie intake and risk of obesity. All else being equal, however, you should favor obtaining your necessary fats from healthier sources rather than trans fats and saturated fats. Note that I used the word necessary fat. So how much fat is necessary and what is excessive?

No one knows the exact amount, but it has been commonly suggested that we should limit our fat intake to no more than 30 percent of our overall calories, although 20 percent may be a better target for many of us.

CARBOHYDRATES & PROTEINS:

Like fats, both carbohydrates and proteins come in various forms and are derived from different sources. Specific types of carbohydrates and proteins found in food have certain advantages and disadvantages. Whenever you look at the nutritional content of a given food or a dietary supplement, you should try to at least get a sense of the type of protein or carbohydrate you are consuming. This is even more important when consuming dietary aids or supplements because these products often contain fat, protein and carbohydrate calories from a variety of sources.

Let's use the example of proteins to illustrate my point. If you want to know what type of protein you are eating, it's best to eat simple foods. Milk, for instance, is an animal source of protein. Beans are also a vegetable source of protein.

The protein sources in packaged foods and nutritional supplements, on the other hand, are much more difficult to determine. If you are consuming, for instance, an energy bar, you would not be able to determine the source of protein by sight. The bar itself is usually just a brownish or whitish color rectangle that does not resemble any of our basic food groups. Who knows where the calories are coming from? Therefore, you will have to look at the ingredients label on the wrapper.

CARBOHYDRATES:

It's time to cover the basic sources of carbohydrates as well as some important caveats to consider.

Carbohydrates are considered to be either **complex** or **simple**. A complex carbohydrate is made up of a combination of simple forms of carbohydrates. The simple forms of carbohydrates are often called "sugars" while the complex forms are often called "starches".

Simple carbohydrates are *generally sweet* and can be found in *fruits and simple sugars such as honey and maple syrup.*

Complex carbohydrates are found in *whole grains* (including breads, pastas and cereals,) *legumes and some vegetables* including potatoes and spinach.

➢ For packaged products, review the list of ingredients section of the nutrition label. The ingredients are generally arranged in a descending order from the most abundant to the least. Keep in mind that "simple" and "complex" are not going to be listed. And, generally speaking, whole foods will be hard to find.

- Examples of simple sugars are: sucrose, glucose, galactose, fructose and lactose
- Examples of complex carbohydrates are: whole grains, flours and vegetable starches

One important trait of complex carbohydrates is that they lead to a more steady level of blood sugar when consumed compared to simple carbohydrates or sugars. In general, the complex forms are better for storage and for future energy needs. Simple carbohydrates have the ability to raise blood sugar levels more quickly and therefore are best for more immediate energy demands.

Eating some complex carbohydrates several hours before a vigorous activity or exercise will often ensure than you will have an adequate energy supply during your workout. On the other side, having a simple carbohydrate may be better for those who want a "pick me up" immediately before or during exercise.

Fortunately our bodies usually have enough energy reserves that we don't need to worry too much about eating carbohydrates before mild or moderate exercise, if we eat a balanced diet. Supplementing and adding carbohydrates becomes more important for athletes and those who participate in demanding exercise as well as individuals who do not consume adequate amounts of this nutrient from their diets.

PROTEINS:

Like fats and carbohydrates, it's also important to analyze the sources of proteins. For instance, different proteins have different *bioavailability.* Protein bioavailability refers to how well your body utilizes a given protein source. Proteins with high bioavailability can be used more completely by the body and are often good for individuals who want to build and maintain muscle mass, such as body builders, or those who frequently exercise.

➤ Examples of protein with higher bioavailability include:
  • Proteins from animal sources such as milk (often called whey), eggs and meat
➤ Examples of proteins with lower bioavailability include:
  • Proteins from vegetable sources such as soy protein or nuts

BALANCING YOUR CALORIES:

➤ A good rule of thumb to assist you in obtaining a balanced diet is to consume approximately:

  ✓ 50% of total calories from carbohydrates
  ✓ 30% of total calories from proteins
  ✓ 20% of total calories from fats

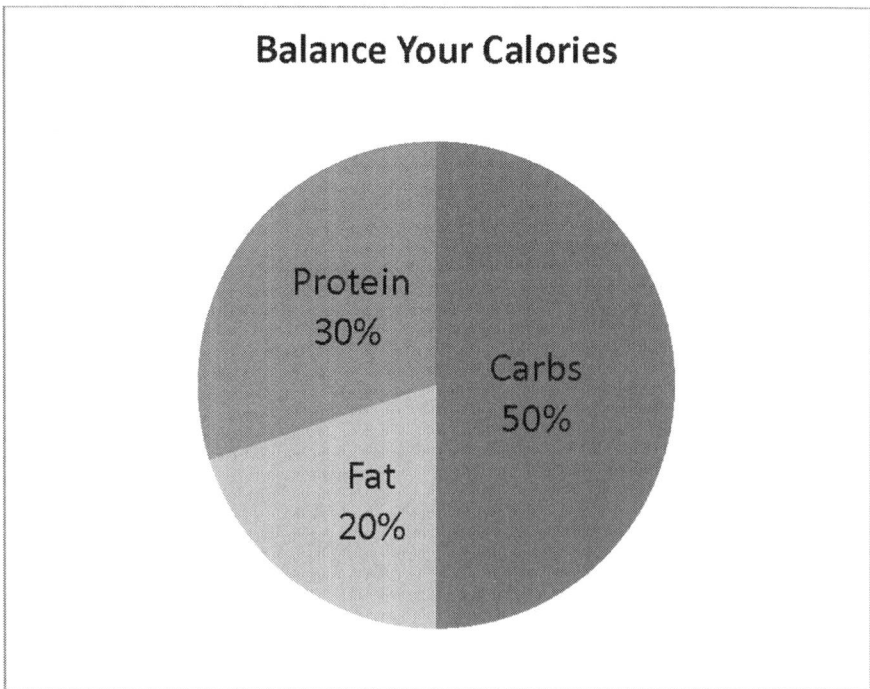

While we cannot say with certainty what the perfect ratio should be, this distribution of calories will likely work well for most adults. That is, this list is not meant to be a hard and fast rule, but rather a rough guide. For example, let's say that you calculate your average daily calorie intake at 2000 calories a day and figure that more than 50% of these calories are from fat. In this case, we can see that you would want to reduce your calories from fat and increase either your proteins, carbohydrates or both.

In the opposite case, let's say your daily calorie consumption matched your required caloric needs, but your fat intake was only 5%. Here, you would want to increase your fat calories while reducing the intake of other calorie sources.

The information contained here and elsewhere throughout this book will help you put together a balanced diet, and the summary plan provided to you later will focus on total calorie consumption, especially during the early stages. Because the program is progressive, you will use some of your acquired knowledge to ensure proper balance as you move through each step of the Healthy 4 program. This involves acute awareness of the foods that you eat and assessment of important nutritional content such as the percentage of proteins, carbohydrates and fats.

CHAPTER FOUR:
BARRIERS TO A PROPER DIET

I have previously mentioned, on several occasions, that paying attention to our calorie consumption is very important. I have also suggested that this allows us to improve our awareness of overconsumption. So what is it exactly that drives us towards overconsumption in the first place? This question has no one simple answer. But we can examine some of the reasons since it is important for us to understand all the pertinent issues before we can proceed with formulating a diet plan. Once we examine and understand the actual forces that cause us to abuse food, we will improve our ability to control these forces and put them to work for us, rather than against us.

A common cause of overconsumption is anxiety. How many of us have been stressed about something in our life and found ourselves headed to the refrigerator? I venture to say that just about everyone does this from time to time. So what is it about stress that can lead to over consumptive behavior?

Anxiety often leads to depression, helplessness and a loss of self-control, which can be contributing factors in a variety of eating disorders. Additionally, this loss of control will often worsen our anxiety and a perpetual cycle can ensue:

Mood Swings → Anxiety

Fatigue

Depression

Diet
Changes

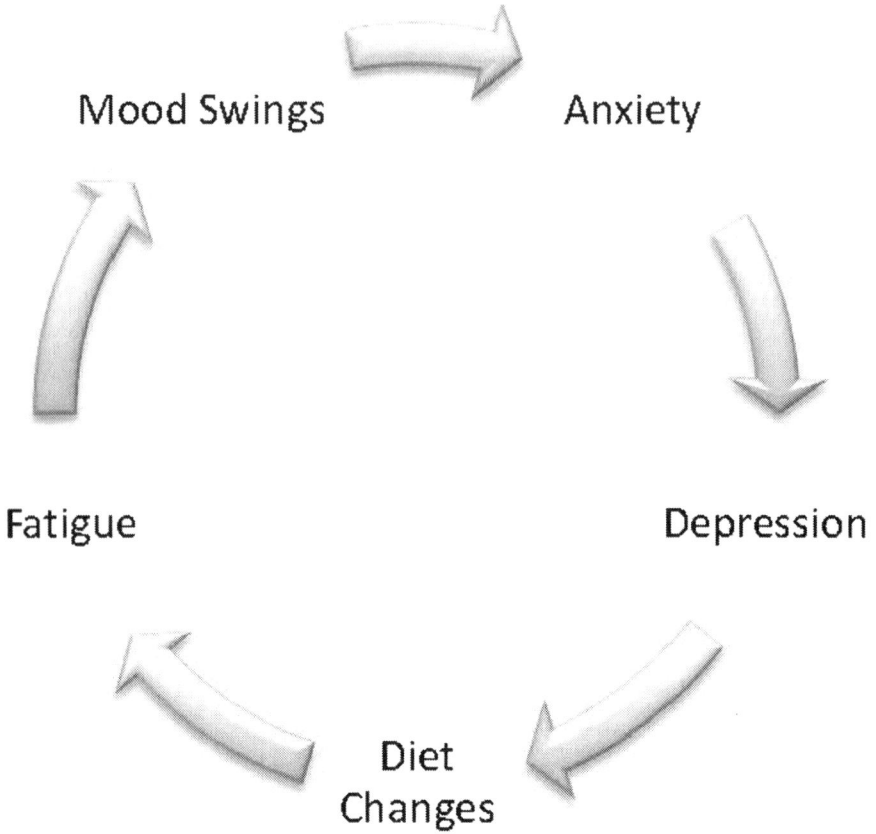

The relationship between anxiety and diet reminds us of the central theme of the Healthy 4 program which states that four dependent key components (diet, exercise, stress reduction and spirituality) control our health and well-being. Thus, by reducing our stress and anxiety, we remove one of the root causes of overeating. You will see that incorporating stress reduction and dieting together not only makes dieting easier, but substantially improves your health over all.

Stress, as we know, can be attributed to many factors such as financial trouble, relationship problems and work related issues. One of the keys to improving our diet is to first *acknowledge* that we feel stress as it occurs.

Next we need to *understand* what exactly is causing our anxiety or stress. In some cases it may be an easily identifiable stressor such as a relationship problem or a recent job loss. However, other times it may be harder to pinpoint or more pervasive, such as feelings of generalized anxiety, which can be due to a medical disorder in certain cases.

Once we acknowledge the presence of a particular stress and understand what's causing it, we'll then be able to apply a variety of stress reduction techniques which may include deep breathing, biofeedback, exercising and meditation among others. We will discuss these coping methods and several more in detail in the section on stress management. For now, just understand that these techniques will help us control our eating habits and improve our diet.

So how do we know if stress is leading us to overeat? Well, besides acknowledgement, an excellent place to start is by monitoring your normal calorie intake, which you are familiar with already. Ask yourself how much you usually eat at one setting and how often.

Obviously, you may not be fully aware of everything you eat at the beginning of the diet plan. It does take some trial and error to figure out how much you need to consume in order to maintain your ideal body weight due to variations in your body's metabolism that occur with dieting and exercise. Over time however, your body will reach a steady state, making it easier to assess your calorie requirements.

Whenever you recognize that anxiety, rather than normal physiological cues, is what is driving you to eat, you must **prescribe** yourself something. No that doesn't mean I want you to self medicate! On the contrary, what I mean is to replace the urge to eat with something else, instead of simply restricting your food intake.

For example, many doctors commonly ask their patients to quit smoking because it's bad for them. Health care providers know all too well that stopping a habit that involves a strong urge can be extremely difficult, especially without replacing that habit with something else.

The individual who is trying to give up an unhealthy activity such as smoking will have a better chance of success if he or she replaces their cigarettes with another object or activity such as chewing gum or a new hobby. In fact, this is why people who quit smoking often eat more, because they are subconsciously replacing food for their cigarettes (which I do not recommend, by the way.)

Some common things to prescribe yourself rather than food during times of stress are:

- ✓ Exercise
- ✓ Water: sometimes thirst is a trigger for eating; drinking a glass of water may curb your appetite
- ✓ A creative hobby or interest: drawing, painting or writing are good ways to refocus your concentration away from food
- ✓ Meditation
- ✓ Yoga
- ✓ Solve a riddle or do a jigsaw puzzle
- ✓ Read a magazine or good book
- ✓ Take a short walk or go outside
- ✓ Organize something: clean the garage or closet, arrange your picture or music albums
- ✓ Talk to a friend, spouse or family member

There are a number of things you can prescribe yourself as a replacement for food in times of stress. Whatever the prescription, you may find that these activities do more than suppress the urge to eat. They may reduce your anxiety level as well by occupying your mind with a productive activity, shifting your focus away from a particular stressor.

A quick word of caution about chewing gum: while, at times this may help substitute for food, the mechanical act of chewing can actually signal the production of certain enzymes and proteins which can in turn lead to hunger. If you must chew or eat something, you may be better off by allowing yourself to snack on something low in calories such as carrot sticks, celery or rice cakes.

Stress is just one of the enemies of a proper diet and healthy eating practices. The next barrier to a proper diet can be blamed on our so called "westernized" culture. What do I mean by this? Unfortunately, we tend to be a society of excess and that is reflected in the portions of food we consume. In the United States, it is not uncommon to be served meals at restaurants and at home that may be several times larger than what is normal in other countries around the world.

Furthermore, many of the foods that we eat are very high in calories due to the extra fats and carbohydrates used to prepare or accent our food. If one is fortunate enough to travel overseas, this excess becomes very apparent when we are served more reasonable food portions, which are clearly smaller than those back home. Even fatty foods and those high in calories are served in limited portion sizes in many other regions around the globe. At first glance, it may feel strange or even unacceptable to us that we receive so little food compared to what we are accustomed to in our industrialized world. These are not necessarily poverty stricken countries where food is a scarce resource. In many affluent countries, people consume much less food than we do. This is manifested in the citizenry, too, where individuals generally have a lower body mass and lower incidence of heart disease as compared to those in the United States.

So what are we to do, when, everywhere we go, things appear to be "supersized" or provide "extra value?" One answer is to **STOP** for a moment and reflect on our fundamental rule:

WHAT WE CONSUME SHOULD BE NO MORE THAN WHAT IS REQUIRED!

Let me give you a quick hypothetical example. Let's assume that you base your diet on 1800 calories per day. For breakfast, you pour yourself a bowl of cereal and a glass of orange juice, which certainly sounds like a sensible meal. However, for lunch you decide to purchase the value meal at your local fast food establishment because it is a "better deal." So, you end up eating 3 cheeseburgers instead of one. If you were to stick to your diet plan, you probably would be done eating for the day since you have likely exceeded your caloric limits. Chances are that you will be starving by dinner time, however, and it's doubtful you would be able to refrain from dinner, thereby sabotaging the diet entirely.

The message here is simple: Avoid eating high calorie meals or large portion sizes. A healthy diet involves consuming smaller, more frequent meals throughout the day, which helps to reduce hunger. The reduction in hunger from smaller meals can be attributed to a healthier blood sugar profile and a decreased storage capacity of the digestive tract.

Our stomach is comprised of elastic tissue that has the capacity to expand over time if we continually overeat. This can cause a viscous cycle, where we need to eat larger and larger quantities of food to feel satisfied. In fact, many people undergo bariatric surgery in an attempt to decrease the capacity of their stomachs. Unfortunately, the effectiveness of these surgeries will often decrease overtime, unless the root cause of the overconsumption is eliminated. Just remember, despite our current cultural trend towards excess, you must avoid this over consumptive behavior and constantly remind yourself that eating smaller portions leads to healthier eating habits and a smaller stomach.

While developing into a culture of material excess, we have simultaneously managed also to evolve into a society of sedentary beings. In fact, we are more inactive now compared to any other period in our history. It is ironic that our culture's quest for greater mobility has actually led us to a state of physical inactivity. Other than the time we may spend on occasional exercise, think about the enormous amount of time we spend sitting during daily commutes, emails, internet use, phone calls and at home.

For many of us, our sedentary life has increased exponentially, leaving little room to efficiently burn calories throughout the day. This certainly makes it more challenging for us to live a healthy lifestyle. Never the less, technology is here to stay and the days of hunting and gathering our food are long gone. Thus, we must try to achieve a healthy body through diet now more than ever.

Restrictions of time and barriers to access are yet other deterrents to a healthy diet. One way to combat this problem is to pack your own lunch or carry healthy snacks or supplements with you. For instance, if you find that your choices at work are limited to unhealthy, fast food or pot luck meals that contain artery hardening fried foods, it would behoove you to BYOF (bring your own food)! As I have suggested, nutrition bars or a meal prepared from home would likely be a much better alternative in this case.

It's important to reiterate that not all nutritional and dietary supplements are made equal. Let's look at protein bars. As you know by now, these are made from a variety of sources of protein but they may also have a large amount of calories from other sources. To pick the right supplement or nutrition bar, you must understand your dietary goals and apply some of the information that we have already discussed.

For instance, if you are training for a 10 kilometer race, your primary need is to increase your energy level with carbohydrates and high quality protein. On the other hand, if your goal is weight reduction, you are seeking a well-balanced, lower calorie supplement to curb your hunger. In either case, it is important to purchase the right nutritional supplement that best fits your goals. As with all packaged foods, you need to read the information on the back of the wrapper or container.

In particular, some of the specific things you should assess when choosing a nutritional bar, drink or powder are as follows:

✓ Look at the serving size and number of calories. Even supplements of similar size can vary greatly in number of calories.

✓ Look at the percentages of fats, carbohydrates and proteins.

✓ Analyze the type of carbohydrates to determine if they are simple or complex. Simple sugars or carbohydrates like sucrose are good for activities requiring short bursts of energy; complex carbohydrates are better for everyday snacking because these calories help sustain activities requiring endurance. Complex carbohydrates also tend to help us maintain a steadier blood sugar level while simple carbohydrates cause wider variations in blood sugar levels.

✓ Analyze protein sources: are they from animal or vegetable sources? Consider their bioavailability, which is the measure of how efficiently our bodies can utilize the food source. Foods with high bioavailability are mostly used by our bodies for our nutritional needs while those that are low in bioavailability are not as available for our body's vital processes.

✓ Check for other ingredients including vitamins and minerals.

While it is neither practical nor often possible to review everything on the nutritional labels, this basic understanding will go a long way towards improving your diet and nutrition. For a more in depth look at health supplements, you will need to investigate other sources. You can start with our website at Healthy4.com. For now, the information that you have is sufficient to allow you to make more informed decisions about food and the basic food supplements that you will commonly encounter.

Another barrier to proper diet may come from our own attitudes and perceptions. For example, some may feel it is too time consuming or too restrictive to their lifestyle to monitor their diet closely. Others may have had poor results with previous diets and are discouraged. Many others have experienced the "yo-yo" effect, meaning that weight loss and gain fluctuates significantly. While this often occurs with new diets, it more often leads to frustration and ultimately a lack of interest in continuing with their plan. To combat these negative feelings and experiences we must change our way of thinking when it comes to dieting.

This is where our fourth health component, **spirituality**, can help. This major component of health can be defined as a willingness to place someone or something in high regard. It involves keeping our own egos in check while we devote our time or energy for the good of another. So what's this got to do with dieting you may ask? Plenty! Just bear with me for a moment, as I hope to show you that spirituality has everything to do with a healthy diet and lifestyle.

Although a sense of self esteem is an important motivating factor, sense of others is equally important. When we improve our diet and our well-being, it improves the health of others as well. Let's examine this underappreciated fact a bit closer. Eating well and maintaining a healthy diet helps to prevent many diseases such as heart disease, stroke, diabetes and certain cancers. In fact, research has indicated that more than 50 percent of diseases causing death are potentially preventable. Therefore, you have the power to live longer and improve your wellness.

Your family and friends will obviously benefit from your increased vitality and longevity. Society also has much to gain. By preserving our individual health, we reduce the burden of preventable disease, conserve valuable health care resources and improve access to care for those who are less fortunate. What a simple yet effective way to contribute to the benefit of mankind!

A tip to counteract negative dietary perceptions involves a technique that we will discuss in more detail in the stress management section of the program. It involves practicing positive internal monologues, which over time facilitate changes in thought and behavior. For instance, we should *never view dieting as a restriction or limitation*. This tends to reinforce negative feelings and reduces one's resolve. *Instead, our diet should be thought of as empowering and liberating*, in the sense that it has the potential to open doors to wellness that would otherwise not exist.

Another negative perception people sometimes have is that dieting is a temporary means to an end, rather than an end itself. To elucidate the difference, consider two different individuals: one individual approaches dieting as a means to lose 20 pounds before an important event such as a wedding. The other approaches diet as a lifelong process to improve health. In the former case, dieting becomes a short term restriction to achieve a finite goal, a quick fix that often leads to "yo-yo" dieting. In the latter case, dieting becomes a way of life which promotes longevity.

The last diet barrier to consider has to do with the belief that dieting is somehow a separate component or problem from other important aspects of our life. This is in direct conflict with the premise of the Healthy 4 program which teaches us that a healthy diet cannot be attained in isolation. Rather, dieting is part of an integrated system of healthy living. As we have said, our overall health is driven by four major factors that interact with one another in a directly proportional manner. In other words, strengthening one of these components leads to a reciprocal improvement in the other components and vice versa. Thus, improper exercise and physical inactivity, for example, can also be a barrier to proper diet.

The link between exercise and diet may seem someone elusive at first, but it should come as no surprise after illustrating a few of their more obvious cause and effect relationships. First, it is most clear perhaps, that one's diet can significantly affect exercise both positively and negatively. Without proper nutrition, exercise becomes exceedingly more difficult. From the other side, exercise endurance is enhanced with optimal nutrition.

Next, poor exercise or a lack of activity can lead to digestive tract problems. In a hospital setting, many patients who are on prolonged bed rest can develop a condition called an Ileus. This occurs when the movement of food through the digestive tract becomes significantly reduced or absent, leading to nausea, vomiting and malnutrition. Early treatment of this condition is physical therapy and walking exercises which help stimulate the digestive tract.

Another more common negative effect of physical inactivity on digestive tract function is indigestion and heartburn. Many people who sit or lay down immediately after eating can develop stomach pain and bloating. So, in addition to modifying the foods we consume, we must also increase our physical activity for proper digestion. This is why many people prefer to take a nice walk after a meal rather than sitting.

On the other hand, strenuous activity or vigorous exercise immediately after a meal will have a counter-productive effect and may lead to nausea or cramps and should be avoided. Remember also that eating large portion sizes will often lead directly to heartburn, lethargy and physical inactivity. Thus, moderation is the key.

Physical inactivity and poor exercise also cause a reduction in metabolism and acutely lowers the body's energy requirement. Unfortunately our dietary habits and our hunger response adapt more slowly to inactivity causing a pattern of overconsumption that can lead to obesity over time. In particular, individuals with disabilities and chronic injuries are prone to these maladaptive consumption patterns.

In my practice of medicine, I have cared for many patients who have sustained injury or disease which has limited their ability to exercise. I personally know the challenges these conditions present. Many times patients develop anxiety, stress and depression, exacerbating the problem. It is not uncommon for persons with certain disabilities to feel a sense of hopelessness and an inability to maintain body weight. While many times, the result is overeating, in other cases, feelings of depression can lead to loss of appetite, poor nutrition and unintended weight loss. Thus, we need to return to our dietary constant for a moment:

THE AMOUNT CONSUMED MUST EQUAL THE AMOUNT THAT WE NEED

This equation often takes on increased significance in cases of physical disability and injury. Thus, a specific chapter covering disability and adapting to change is included in the upcoming exercise section of this program. At this point, the message to those faced with physical afflictions or chronic injury and pain is that you can overcome difficult challenges and find wellness with the right mindset and a good plan.

CHAPTER FIVE:
HEALTHY HABITS AND WEIGHT LOSS

In our final chapter on diet, we will discuss healthy eating habits and review methods to avoid overconsumption. For many people, one of the most desirable effects of dieting is weight loss. Thus, we will also approach the topic of body mass and weight reduction. At the end of the chapter, we will put our concepts into action with a diet summary plan that pulls all of the information together.

As we know, hunger is a complex bodily response that can be triggered by a variety of stimuli. These cues to hunger may be internal or external. External cues include a familiar or inviting aroma or the appetizing appearance of a dessert tray. Many chefs are masters at knowing how to present food in a way that is visually appealing.

It is very important to recognize these external cues to hunger so we can prevent them from influencing our important dietary considerations. Specifically, we must always consider four things in a dietary plan. I refer to these decisions as the *Big Four of Dieting.* These are the *Why, When, What and How* decisions. That is to say, you must always ask yourself four main questions when following any diet plan or before consuming *any* food or drink. These questions are:

```
1  • Why Am I Eating?
2  • When Should I Eat?
3  • What Should I Eat?
4  • How Much Should I Eat?
          • BIG  4
```

The first and most important question to ask your self is why am I eating? Ask why you are eating *every time* you consider consuming any food or drink. As it pertains to an individual diet plan, the answer is simple: We eat to obtain the necessary balanced nutrition that is required for good health. We should *not* eat to satisfy hunger! As I have said, hunger can be triggered by many cues that are both internal and external. For instance, we know how the smell of warm apple pie or the sight of hot fudge ice cream can make our mouths water and cause us to consume food. When this happens (as it frequently does,) you must consider your dietary goals and whether this food is appropriate to consume under your individual diet plan. If the answer to that question is no, then you know what the answer is already: *Don't eat it.*

I am not saying that your food should not be satisfying. Of course, it's ok to enjoy the food we eat so long as it fits with our overall dietary goals. However, seeking pleasure and comfort in food is a common cause of over consumption as well as obesity and must be avoided. Again, we will review techniques to assist you with this in a little while. For the time being, just remember that you control your own food intake; food does not control you!

At other times, the answer to "why am I eating?" is an internal cue. These can be much less obvious. Recall our discussion of anxiety as a cause of over-consumption. Eating when we feel nervous or anxious will not control either of these problems. In fact, eating will probably make things worse. Once you recognize that certain internal cues have nothing to do with nutritional hunger, you can avoid overconsumption and deal with these unresolved conflicts appropriately. We will describe methods to reduce anxiety later in the stress management section.

Lastly, our internal cue to hunger may truly be a normal physiologic response, such as a decreasing blood sugar concentration. In this case, we will need to consume some food to restore normal energy reserves. However, we must be careful not to over consume food in this case. Rather, we need to reduce our hunger in healthier ways.

As far as the other three questions of when, what and how much to consume, we already addressed these in earlier chapters. The answers to all the questions are based on your daily calorie consumption goals, while keeping in mind a balanced diet.

An important healthy eating practice is to **slow down**! We are often in a rush due to our hectic lifestyle. A reflection of this can be seen in our hurried eating behavior at the dinner table. Try to eat and drink your meals much slower. One benefit will be an improvement in the taste and enjoyment of food. Chewing slowly and taking routine breaks from eating allows you to savor your food and fully appreciate its unique flavors. To completely understand this rationale, I will use a phrase that is commonly applied in the study of economics, which is "the law of diminishing returns."

We all know that the first few bites of food are the most enjoyable. If, during a meal, you begin to sense that the food is losing its flavor or satisfaction, then you have already experienced this law of diminishing returns. It's difficult to detect this taste change when you eat in a rapid manner.

The goal should be to avoid this phenomenon from occurring in the first place. By the time you start to notice a change in the taste of your food, it's probably too late and you have consumed too much. The key is to finish your meal at a point where the last bite is just as good as the first bite, before the law of diminishing returns occurs. This way, you enjoy more of your food and avoid overeating.

There is another, more scientific, reason why eating slowly can reduce your overall consumption. When we eat too quickly, we do not give our body enough time to digest our food and it is digestion that helps signal our brain to decrease our hunger level. For instance, our blood sugar concentration is an important physiologic cue that signals our hunger response. Hunger is initiated by low blood sugar levels, while higher blood sugar levels have the opposite inhibitory effect on hunger. Eating slowly allows us to digest and absorb some of our nutrients before we are done with our meal. This will help elevate blood sugar and reduce hunger.

Thus, you can decrease or stop your hunger with less food. If you eat too fast however, your body will not have time to absorb the nutrient chemicals needed to reduce your hunger level. In this situation, we rely on other, more mechanical methods for reducing hunger and sensing fullness. This involves a stomach stretch reflex that signals your brain that you are full.

Recall for a moment our gas tank analogy from the first chapter. Filling the tank completely is not necessary to get you from point A to point B. Nor is it necessary to obtain adequate nutrition and maintain a healthy diet. Unless you have had previous gastric surgery, eating until you actually feel "full" means that you are probably eating too much food at one time. In order to avoid overconsumption you may frequently need to remind yourself to slow down if you are in the habit of eating quickly, especially if your blood sugar is too low or you have a strong hunger response prior to consuming your meal.

As I have alluded to previously, you should have some desire to eat more when you are finished with a meal, rather than feel full. It is very important to retrain your brain and body to walk away from the table with some room to comfortably eat more if you wanted. It takes a little time to find the right balance between walking away hungry and consuming just enough food. Repeating the following mantra before each meal may help:

ALWAYS UNDER NEVER OVER

The long version is: I *can always eat more when I under eat,* but I *can never eat less once I over eat.*

Another disadvantage of eating too fast is that it may cause a large surge of carbohydrates and simple sugars to enter your blood stream. For instance, a condition called "reactive hypoglycemia" characterized by rapid swings in blood sugar can occur after consuming a large meal. As we know, digestion is a complex and finely tuned process that can be used to our advantage in some cases but cause problems in other cases. In order to understand reactive hypoglycemia, we need to examine some basic physiology. Don't worry, I promise to keep it simple.

Most of us are familiar with the hormone insulin, which is used exogenously by those with diabetes mellitus. Insulin helps regulate our blood sugar level throughout the day by lowering the level of sugar in our blood stream. When we eat foods such as carbohydrates or sugars, our bodies produce more of the hormone, which in turn helps deliver the sugar into our organs and cells. If our blood sugar is low, our body decreases its insulin production to help normalize our sugar level. If our blood sugar is too high (such as after a meal) insulin is increased to help lower the sugar level to a more normal state.

Diabetic people often have a problem with high blood sugar because they have too little insulin or the body doesn't recognize the insulin properly, which causes the blood sugar level to remain high. Reactive hypoglycemia, however, is a temporary and direct result of eating too much or too fast. Basically, the large amount of sugar from the food enters the blood stream too quickly, which causes an abnormally high spike of insulin. As all of you are now aware, insulin lowers the blood sugar level, and because there is too much insulin present, blood sugar becomes abnormally low despite recently eating.

When blood sugar becomes too low we can feel weak or lethargic and our ability to concentrate becomes reduced. But, again, low blood sugar can stimulate appetite. So eating or drinking too much or too fast can lead to inactivity and perpetuate our desire to continue eating. It is a viscous cycle but one that can be prevented by eating more slowly.

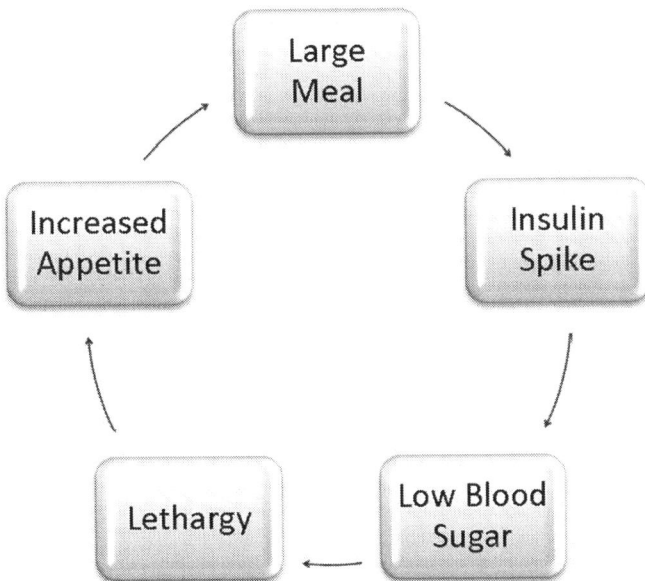

If you, like most of us, are someone who has little free time to sit down to a relaxing two hour meal, you may not be able to eat much slower but you can still reduce the amount you eat at one time. You will have to consume small, quick snacks or meals more frequently throughout the day. For example, it only takes a couple of minutes to have an apple, a nutrition bar or half of a sandwich if you are busy. This saves time and helps to prevent low blood sugar, which can negatively affect your work as well as make you hungrier.

Regardless of our time schedules, we should all try to eat smaller, more frequent snacks rather than two or three large meals. This is another healthy pattern that can keep our sugar level more constant and prevent undesirable rapid changes in blood sugar. So, to get back to our gas tank analogy, we can eat small, more frequent meals, keeping our "tanks" fairly empty but preventing us from running out of fuel.

Another simple method of preventing over consumption is to add foods low in caloric content. For example, substituting a chicken breast for a cheese burger or eating carrots or celery sticks instead of potato chips is a good place to start. One of the benefits of consuming low calorie snacks is that you can eat a larger volume of food compared to a higher calorie snack. As we have discussed previously, however, if something says "reduced calorie" or "reduced fat," you should not simply ingest more without regard to your consumption goals.

Unfortunately, some people on diets become too caught up in minimizing a specific source of calories. You will often see this with certain fad diets such as the "low carb" or "low fat" diets. Instead, we know that the focus should be on overall calorie consumption within the framework of a proper balance.

On a per-weight basis, a gram of fat does indeed contain more calories than a gram of carbohydrate or protein. The number of calories per gram of fat, protein and carbohydrate are as follows:

> ➢ **One Gram of Fat = 9 Calories**
> ➢ **One Gram of Protein = 4 Calories**
> ➢ **One Gram of Carbohydrate = 4 Calories**

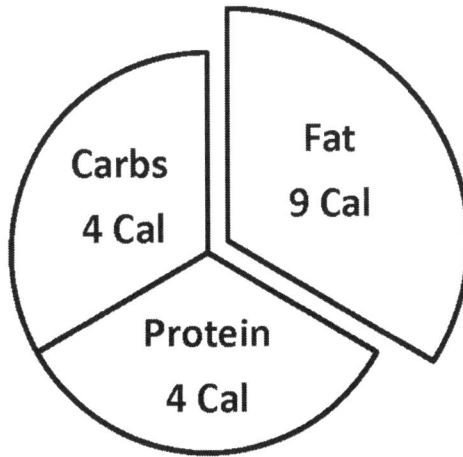

As we can see, fat has more than twice the calories as protein or carbohydrates on a per weight basis. However, we all know how easy it can be to over consume so called "diet foods" that are low in fat content. While a bag of baked potato chips may have no fat, for example, it is far from zero calories.

The recurring message is this: Don't get fooled by food labels or marketing schemes that suggest something is reduced calories or low in fat. Be the judge for yourself. Consuming certain foods or drinks lower in calories or fats may be a good place to start, especially if you consume too many high calorie foods now. However, you must always remember to monitor each meal closely no matter what you eat.

So, let's review our healthy diet habits before moving forward with our diet plan.

> ➢ Avoid eating until full. You should still have some appetite remaining when you are finished with a meal. Remember, *"always less never more!"*
> ➢ Eat small portions. AVOID *"super sizing"* or *"extra value"* menus!
> ➢ Eat more frequently during the day rather than relying on one or two large meals.
> ➢ Don't wait until your hunger is strong before you eat. It is much easier to control yourself if your hunger is mild.
> ➢ SLOW DOWN when you eat. Chew slowly and concentrate on the taste of each and every bite or sip.

➢ Avoid eating as a reflex to hunger. Assess for any abnormal cues to hunger such as anxiety or whether there is an external cue such as a pleasant smell or sight.

➢ Consume lower or low calorie foods and drinks.

➢ Drink plenty of water during the day to avoid dehydration. Thirst can be confused for hunger.

➢ Drink mostly water and avoid soft drinks or other high calorie juices.

➢ Try snacking *before* a meal and do "ruin your appetite" with a healthy snack.

➢ When dining out, **forget** about the traditional courses. It's okay to eat just one or two different courses or several small healthy appetizers rather than a full entrée.

➢ Pack your own lunch or carry nutrition bars and supplements with you.

➢ NEVER eat from buffets or all you can eat menus!

➢ Focus on basic foods and simple meals. If you don't know what's on your plate don't eat it.

➢ DON'T feel guilty if you don't clear your plate. STOP eating once you meet your dietary goals. Overconsumption wastes much more food over the long run.

➢ DO count your calories!

➢ DON'T let hunger guide you. Set a daily calorie consumption goal and stick to it!

➢ Eat a well-balanced diet including fruits, grains, green leafy vegetables, low fat protein such as chicken breast or fish, and low fat dairy products.

➢ When eating healthy foods assign them positive thoughts; for example, think of toast without butter as "natural" or "healthy" rather than "dry" or "plain.

➢ When eating unhealthy foods assign them negative thoughts. For example think of fried food as "artery clogging" or "greasy" rather than "good" or "tasty".

➢ Obtain most of your daily fats from unsaturated, non-trans fat sources such as canola oil, vegetable oil, olive oil or walnut oil.

➢ Never eat before bedtime or lay sedentary after you eat. Try a small walk instead.

➢ Last but not least, focus on food preparation and minimize your use of high calorie condiments, spreads and dressings!

WEIGHT LOSS AND IDEAL BODY WEIGHT:

If one of your dietary goals is to lose weight, this is best done as a gradual and steady drop until your ideal body weight is achieved. You will use the information from your dietary consumption log book to help establish a gradual weight loss. For example, if you find that you consume 1900 calories per day, but you are still unable to lose weight, it will not help to base your consumption on a typical 2000 calorie per day diet (such as that established by the RDA). In this case, you will have to reduce your caloric intake and/or advance the exercise component of this program to help you achieve your goals.

On the other hand, if you have a fairly normal activity level and your average intake is 3500 calories per day, you will have a lot of working room. In this case you will be able to lose weight sufficiently by reducing your calories.

You don't need to focus on an actual number of pounds to lose. If you prefer, you can try losing a pound or two a week for example, rather than establishing a finite number such as a 20 pound weight loss over a certain period of time. Setting your mind on one large number when we are motivated will not help us when we are feeling anxious or deprived. Focusing on a single isolated number is often unrealistic and not useful.

What's important is setting small goals and frequent progress reminders rather than an isolated, arbitrary goal of 50 or 100 pounds of weight loss for example. It's okay to keep these considerations in the back of your mind, but more importantly continue to monitor small steps and daily or weekly objectives. For instance, what if you only lose 10 pounds over 3 months despite setting a goal of 20 pounds? Does this mean you've failed? Of course not! In this case, you are likely healthier already and have made positive gains in your goal towards an ideal body weight and a healthy life.

Furthermore, we know that dieting and weight control is a lifestyle that doesn't end if you gain weight or have periodic setbacks. Every little bit of improvement counts in your quest to become healthier.

What is the "ideal body weight"? Every person probably has a different perception of what their own should be. However, there are guidelines that have been established that use your current weight and height to help define ideal body weight and obesity. To find out more about your ideal body weight, go to www.Healthy4.com.

There are several ways to measure body fat percentage and the ideal body weight. Although each method has its advantages and disadvantages, the body mass index (BMI) is a quick reference with established guidelines that are based on your weight and height.

Keep in mind that we are not all made equal and body weight does depend on several important factors such as your gender, muscle mass and age. Nevertheless, calculating your body mass index or BMI can be a very helpful tool, since a high BMI has been correlated with many life threatening diseases and serious health problems. Below I will provide you with some quick definitions of body type based on BMI.

Quick BMI Reference Chart:

BODY MASS INDEX (BMI)	BODY HABITUS
BETWEEN 19 & 25	IDEAL BODY WEIGHT
BETWEEN 25 & 30	OVER WEIGHT
GREATER THAN 30	OBESE
GREATER THAN 40	MORBIDLY OBESE

Again, you can find out your BMI and body type by going to our web site: www. Healthy4.com and following the "health resources" link on the home page.

Some of you may be a little frightened to check on your body type or may feel discouraged by the information that you obtain. Don't get too caught up in the numbers, especially at the beginning. The BMI chart, just like your body weight, is a tool that helps us to establish guidelines and will help you monitor your progress.

These measurements do not exist to make you feel bad about yourself or give you the sense that you are failing in your efforts. While it is important that you use all available diet and weight control tools at your disposal, you need to keep in mind that they are only reference points that allow you to monitor progress at various stages. So if the weight scale or BMI calculator gives you a number you don't want to see, don't fret. The good news is that with a little determination and by following the principles outlined in this book you are already on your road to a healthier you.

As I have said, measuring your body weight or counting your calories are simply tools and you should not define success or failure by these alone. Definitely use them to your advantage, however, as information is power. Along with tracking your progress by the numbers, you should monitor yourself visually as well. What I mean is simply this: *really take a good look at yourself.*

As simple as it sounds, there is a right way and a wrong way to do this. I want you to stand in front of the mirror on a regular basis, at least once a day if not more. Don't be embarrassed by this. Try not to feel uncomfortable or feel that it is somehow vain. It's your body and it is one of God's truly miraculous inventions. There is no such thing as an ugly body. Our body is truly beautiful despite how we or others may make us feel about it.

It may be true that we are overweight or have fatty tissue in areas where we don't want it to exist. It's ok! The main point is to forget those who may pass judgment and try hard to ignore passing judgment on yourself. Despite what anyone says, our bodies are all truly beautiful. It does amazing things each and every day. That should be your mantra. Convince yourself of it because it's true!

Next, forget about perfection or comparison to others. It's fine to admire someone with an attractive physique or become motivated by someone in shape. However, never focus your energy and time trying to look like another person. Although you may feel motivation to diet and exercise by constantly telling yourself you hate the way you look, it goes against the Healthy 4 principle. Furthermore this negative dialogue will ultimately reduce your ability to achieve optimal health. Remember that there are **four** key components to health. True, diet and exercise will help you achieve the shape you want. But pursuing this goal because of envy or constant comparison to others can cause negative self-esteem as well as unnecessary stress that will impede your health.

The correct way to look at yourself is by first loving who you are and your body. Next, improve your health and body for your well-being and the well-being of others. Do not diet and exercise in spite of yourself. In other words, do these things to feel *even* better about yourself. Do it to be healthier and live longer, so that you and those around you can benefit from your success. There is obviously nothing wrong if you feel more attractive when you burn excess fat and improve your shape. In fact, that sense of self accomplishment is also an important part of the process.

From now on, when you look in the mirror, I want you to find things about yourself that are attractive. I also want you to evaluate yourself for areas of self-improvement without being too critical. Only evaluate things that you have the power to improve. For example, if you are shorter than average height or have a noticeable blemish or scar, forget about it. There is no point to that type of assessment. Chances are that you are the only one who is truly concerned about your so-called imperfections anyhow.

On the other hand, if you feel that you can improve your waistline through diet and exercise then definitely go for it and continue to monitor yourself often throughout this process. Remember that you are refining and improving your body shape to improve your health and well-being. As you evaluate your body you should often reaffirm those traits that are particularly attractive to you. This could be your eyes, your smile, the shape of your hands or thighs or whatever it is that stands out to you in a positive way. Remember, beauty is never absolute and no one is perfect. We all possess some attractive features and yet all of us have certain features that we feel are less than desirable.

Once you identify one or two areas of your body that you would like to improve the most, I want you to focus on this area every day and use it to motivate yourself to diet and exercise. I want you to concentrate on this region when you are assessing yourself each day and visualize this actual transformation taking place. Once you have a mental picture, then you go out and do it by applying everything that you will learn in this program.

The key is to think positively about how to improve a certain area and actually see that transformation take place in your mind. This works better than using negative thoughts or statements such as "I hate this part" or "I must get rid of this part." Think about how truly funny it sounds when we make comments like "I hate my butt, I've got to get rid of it!" Do you really want to do that? Now, I don't know about you, but I think most of us would find it really hard to sit without a butt! Again, positive internal monologue is very important to our success.

A more positive affirmation might sound something more like this: "I find my stomach to be one of my stronger physical attributes, but I am going to concentrate on firming my buttocks since this is the area that I feel that I can improve upon the most. I am going to actually see myself improve throughout this process. The change is within me and I am excited about working towards my goals."

I think you get my message. Each and every day you must try to take pride in the fact that you are pursuing your goals. You should engage in positive reaffirmation frequently throughout this process. Never set goals that are too rigid or too far into the future. Rather, allow yourself to feel a sense of accomplishment for any improvement that you make along your journey. You do not become healthy or happy the moment you reach a certain weight or shape.

Rather, your goal is to improve continually, each and every day. In essence, it is the process itself, rather than meeting a single specific goal, that allows you to feel and become a healthier and happier person.

At this point you have multiple methods of monitoring your diet and its success. Some of these ways involve "the numbers" and include monitoring calories, weighing yourself regularly and calculating a BMI. You also have a visual method and understand how to use a constructive monologue to reinforce positive results. Feel free to use all of these methods, since more information leads to knowledge and – as we all know – knowledge is power.

Before we take a look at our diet plan, remember to use as many of the healthy dietary habits and tips as possible and continue to monitor your weight throughout your diet. Remind yourself frequently that establishing a proper diet does not happen overnight, just as our habits do not develop overnight. Therefore, you must approach the act of dieting as a lifestyle. With time and persistence, your efforts will be rewarded handsomely as you notice improved health, energy and happiness. Now that you are armed with the necessary information and knowledge, we can put together our basic diet plan and complete this part of the program.

HEALTHY 4 SUMMARY PLAN FOR DIET:

<u>DAY 1 – 15:</u>

➢ Buy a log book and write down all your calorie consumption for each day

➢ Review the nutritional labels of foods that you eat and drink so you can record your calories and build nutritional awareness

➢ Do **not** change your normal diet during this stage; focus on building nutritional skills and knowledge that you will use later

<u>DAY 16 – 30:</u>

➢ Choose a daily calorie consumption goal and stick to it (use your log book from the first 15 days to help you establish this goal); you may consider 2000 calories per day if you are currently overweight and consume more than this amount

➢ Continue to monitor your calorie intake by using your log book

➢ Use all the healthy eating techniques discussed in this chapter to assist you in maintaining your consumption goals and avoid overeating

➢ Try to eat a balanced diet

<u>DAY 31 – 90:</u>

➢ Begin to monitor your weight loss visually and by the numbers

➢ Continue to monitor your calorie intake by using your log book

➢ Refine your daily calorie consumption goals based on your progress; use this period to make refinements every week to two weeks, if needed

<u>BEYOND DAY 90:</u>

➢ Continue to follow and perfect everything you have learned

FINAL THOUGHTS:

We will be discussing the second major component of the Healthy 4 system, **exercise**, in our next chapter. The combination of both diet and exercise allows us to more efficiently burn calories, maintain body weight and helps to reinforce positive healthy behaviors essential to our future success.

It is important to keep monitoring your diet closely when making significant changes to your activity or exercise program. This is because the increased physiologic demands of exercise not only burns more calories, but requires more calories as well. Thus, if you lose sight of your healthy dietary habits and calorie monitoring during periods of increased exercise, you may actually gain unwanted weight. The way to prevent this from occurring is to always remember the central theme of this program which is to **integrate all four health components together to optimize results.**

Notice that the last segment of the diet summary plan, "beyond 90 days" has been left open ended. This is done as a purposeful reminder to us. As you recall, diets are for life, not for short periods of time. You should expect that you will continually redefine and reshape your diet throughout your life, based on knowledge gained here as well as changes in your own body's needs.

During this last period, beyond 90 days, it is optional to continue to use a written calorie log. While it certainly has merit anytime, it is most useful in the first several months as you learn to modify your diet. Part of this decision will be based on your comfort level and acquired knowledge of the basic food groups. At this point you may have the skills and knowledge to monitor your diet mentally without the need for a written log. Moreover, if you have a setback in the future, you can always return to the written technique.

This section has provided you with the basic concepts and framework that is crucial to the success of any diet. I know that you can improve your health if you adhere to the techniques and recommendations as outlined. You now have the foundation to build a better diet, which is the first piece of the puzzle. By integrating this component with exercise, stress reduction and spirituality you will maximize your health, longevity and overall well-being.

COMPONENT TWO:
EXERCISE

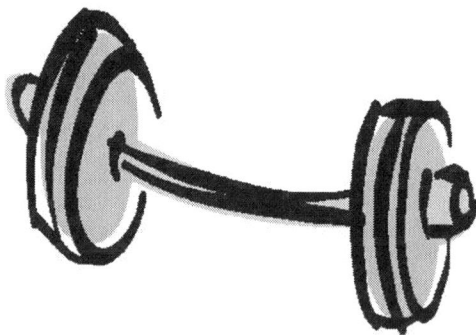

CHAPTER SIX:
INTEGRATING EXERCISE AND DIET

In this section, we will review various types of exercise and their impact on health and well-being. Furthermore, we will explore how exercise, when done properly, influences diet, stress reduction and spirituality to promote exponential health benefits. As with diet, physical fitness should be approached as a way of life, rather than a short term goal, to achieve significant benefits.

I am sometimes asked if it's possible to stay in shape without spending much time on exercise. It is true, as I alluded to during our discussion on diet, that you can maintain your body weight and improve your health by focusing primarily on food consumption. For instance, people who have been afflicted by severe arthritis or even paralysis can still maintain their physique and improve their health by applying the principle:

WHAT WE CONSUME MUST EQUAL THE AMOUNT WE BURN

On the other hand, staying in shape takes on another meaning altogether if we consider our internal organs and blood vessels. It is possible to appear physically healthy on the outside but be "out of shape" on the inside. For instance, a person may have dangerously high cholesterol or high blood pressure, which are known risk factors for cardiovascular disease. We all either know or have heard stories of someone who appeared to be in great shape, yet suffered a heart attack in the prime of his or her life. In some cases this is due to a familial disposition or genetic trait. In others, this may be due to a lack of exercise, smoking or high job stress.

The point is that we can never truly judge how healthy someone is by the way he or she appears. As the saying goes, never judge a book by its cover. The same can be said about our physical shape. Although body habitus is a very strong predictor of health, it is not the only one. The human body is complex and the combination of many risk factors can positively or negatively impact our overall health. Thankfully, many of these factors are modifiable and can be addressed by targeting just a few specific areas. We can decrease our overall risk of illness and improve our health by avoiding certain behaviors and adding new practices to our daily routine.

The premise of this book is that we achieve our optimal health by integrating proper diet, exercise, stress reduction and spirituality into a single program. So, to return to the question, "Is it possible to stay in shape with little or no exercise?" The answer is that you can be healthier through diet alone but you will not achieve total well-being unless you incorporate an exercise program into your life.

Let's revisit our automobile analogy used in the section on diet. In addition to fuel, our cars require routine minor maintenance to optimize their performance and longevity. For example, we often need to change the oil to remove harmful impurities or change the air filter to improve the quality of air intake into the engine. If we neglect these periodic visits, it may cost us a whole lot more in the future. I am sure anyone who has ever experienced a failed transmission or seized engine can attest to that. Major car repairs are not only inconvenient but costly and, sometimes, we realize that the problem cannot be completely reversed.

Similarly, we need to perform routine maintenance on our own bodies to improve its efficiency and reduce damage down the road. Exercise allows us to enhance our performance and helps prevent major work in the future, such as surgery for damaged organs or joints. As a surgeon with more than a decade of patient care experience, I can tell you that, in most cases, our original parts have a better warranty than our replacement parts.

This is not to say that the medical field is not advanced. On the contrary, great accomplishments have been achieved over the last century. The critical point is that despite advances in modern medicine, health care providers will never recreate what nature or God has perfected. Most of us are blessed by health and this gift should be preserved to the best of our ability. We all have the powerful tools at our disposal to improve our own health. Like dieting, exercise is needed to improve our well-being and reduce suffering from disease.

To use another analogy, our health can be viewed as an investment portfolio. In order to limit risk and maximize our returns, we often diversify our funds by allocating them into several different resources. For example, we can apply our funds into several different investments such as annuities, stocks, bonds and real estate. Why do we do this? One good reason is because they all have unique advantages on their own. Moreover, by combining several investments we can limit our losses while maximizing our profits.

Similarly, we should diversify our "health portfolio." Focusing primarily on one component, such as diet, while neglecting others may improve your health to a degree but over the long run this will not provide the necessary synergy to optimize health. Thus, we should combine diet and exercise to improve our overall health and reduce our risk of disease. Ultimately our mission is to integrate all four major components of health into a single program or lifestyle to maximize well-being and enhance longevity.

CHAPTER SEVEN:
BARRIERS TO EXERCISE

There are those of you out there who are eager to participate in healthy activity; however you may feel there are constraints or other limitations that restrict you from incorporating some of these activities into your daily routine. Exercise, in particular, seems to be the health component that is most susceptible to this kind of mindset for several reasons.

First, it is usually perceived as the most time consuming of our Healthy 4 components, and for this reason it is often neglected when time becomes more limited. Second, unlike the other health practices, it is associated with the highest level of exertion, requiring not only mental energy, but physical stamina which, for some, can be challenging.

Next, restriction to access and resources, such as money for gym membership or exercise classes, can limit one's ability to exercise as well. Lastly, some of us are restricted by our lack of knowledge about exercise, such as which activities are best for us and how long we should engage in any activity at one time.

Let's review some of these barriers in greater depth, beginning with time constraints, the most frequently cited reason for neglecting exercise. We are not going to deny that exercise can be time consuming, and some people require more than others. Leading an active or healthy lifestyle does require some time and effort just as most important things in life do.

Some physical activities require more time than others and if you join a gym or class you will have to add in driving, parking, changing, chatting and everything else that goes into it. But all exercise does not require this. In fact, the exercises and techniques provided in this chapter and throughout this book do not require much time at all and by combining several health components together, including exercise, we increase our efficiency and our ability to maximize health, thus saving time overall.

Financial constraints are another barrier to exercise. Since the rise in "getting physical" began several decades ago, gyms and fitness centers have sprung up throughout the country filled with large and sometimes intimidating equipment.

Every few years a new fitness fad brings with it any number of props and equipment, from yoga balls to steppers to fitness bands. If we wanted to, we could spend thousands of dollars a year on working up a sweat. If you have the resources, the time and the energy, there is certainly nothing wrong with any of these. But they are not necessary. For many of us, simple calisthenics and adding more movement to your day is enough to get started and maintain a fitness routine with no financial output at all.

Basic exercise and activity tips for those with limited time or resources include:

1. Take the stairs whenever possible instead of the elevator. You can burn a significant amount of calories per day just by using the stairs, and this is usually faster than waiting for the elevator, anyway.
2. *Don't* look for a good spot in the parking lot or on the street. Try parking your car far away: The walking will be very good for you. There are other advantages as well. First, you avoid the aggravation and stress that comes with circling the lot and dealing with other stressed out drivers. Second, you save time (and gas) since farther parking is quicker to find. Lastly, you'll probably reduce the number of those darn door dings.
3. Take a 5 minute break during the day for sit ups or push ups. These are good musculoskeletal conditioning exercises and relieve stress at the same time. They will also increase your heart rate just enough to burn a handful of calories and give you an energy boost, too.

4. Go for a brisk walk or short jog. Take a few minutes of your day to spend alone or with a friend. Morning walks are enjoyable for their solitude and quiet and prepare your mind for the day ahead. Jogging or walking after work is a good stress reliever and creates a transition between work and home, allowing your mind some time to unwind.

5. When at home, make love, not war. It's healthier for you and your partner. A good argument can certainly get the blood pumping, but the stress that goes with it will outweigh any benefit.

6. Do work outdoors such as gardening or yard work: this has both a physical benefit and a mind-lifting benefit since spending time in natural light lifts the spirit.

7. If you would like to workout at a local fitness club or gym, ask about volunteering in exchange for a free membership or reduced rates.

The last barrier to exercise on our list is fatigue. When tired, it is often difficult to find the motivation to exercise. Exercise performance is also reduced. Extreme fatigue or exhaustion during exercise may increase your susceptibility to the common cold and other communicable diseases, especially if you exercise in a crowded public place. In these extreme cases, it's probably best to avoid strenuous physical activity until you can get plenty of rest. However, most of the time, a little exercise combats fatigue by improving energy levels. This is thought to be the result of certain hormones which are released during exercise, including endorphins and adrenaline.

To combat fatigue, change your exercise time or workout duration. For example, if you are often tired when you exercise after a long day's work, try exercising in the early morning, before work or on your lunch break. You will have more energy at theses times and probably less stress after work since that is one less thing to do at the day's end.

If exercise is leading to fatigue or exacerbating your condition, you may be overtraining. In this case you may need a few days off or, alternatively, you may benefit by changing up your exercise routine. Sometimes just reducing the length of your workouts helps combat overtraining. This is where common sense and listening to your body takes precedent.

Lastly, all exercise programs require commitment and disciple. The key to enduring results is not necessarily how hard you work out during a few isolated sessions, but rather how well you stick to your program. But of course this long term commitment is the basis behind the entire Healthy 4 program and not just the individual exercise component. By the time you have completed this book you will have learned how to begin your quest for a permanently healthier body and mind.

CHAPTER EIGHT:
EXERCISE AND DIET FOR THE INJURED OR DISABLED

I previously stated that proper diet is essential in those with significant physical limitations and chronic injury since activity level is often reduced. However, this does not mean that exercise is any less important. In reality, it is essential for those with physical challenges or limited mobility to help optimize health.

Let's revisit dietary considerations and our constant: The amount consumed should equal the amount used. We know that dietary habits that developed prior to an injury or an affliction must change to reflect an overall decrease in physical activity. Since the amount of activity is often significantly reduced in these situations, so should caloric intake. Of course, this is easier said than done. I have seen many patients with disabilities become frustrated with weight gain due to decreased physical activity. In reviewing diet history, however, it is not uncommon to see consumption patterns that are maladaptive. In some cases, individuals may be eating the same or even more than they did before the disability.

The most common theme that I have heard from patients is that it's very difficult to cut back on calories. But how can anyone blame them? For many of us, even without injury, overeating and dietary habits are problematic. So it is not difficult to imagine the barriers and obstacles of those who are physically challenged. Yet, it is not impossible and I have seen patients overcome enormous challenges. These individuals have achieved incredible accomplishments through pure determination, coupled with a good plan.

Not so long ago I had a patient (we'll call him Bob), visit me at the office. Bob was in his sixties and had suffered from morbid obesity for most of his life. Recall that morbid obesity is a term we use to describe someone who has a body mass index (BMI) greater than 40. What this means is that his health was at very serious risk. I won't give you his exact weight for reasons of patient confidentiality, but I can tell you that he was several times larger than an average person for his given height. To complicate matters greatly, Bob had severe destruction of his joints from wear and tear arthritis. His joint destruction combined with his severe weight problem caused him to be almost entirely sedentary. Although Bob had severe pain and needed his joints replaced, he was very concerned about undergoing surgery as his weight put him at high risk for complications. That day Bob and I sat down and came up with a plan. The plan called for a significant weight reduction and later joint replacement surgery once his obesity was better controlled. We discussed various methods of weight loss and I made a few extra recommendations that day. Before he left the office Bob said something I'll never forget. He said, "See you in six months, doc!" Keep in mind, I have seen many patients over the years with similar challenges and I have heard the phrase, "see you in a few months," too many times to count. What was unique about Bob was not what he said, but how he said it. Despite the great adversity he faced, he looked at me and I could see in his eyes, and hear in his voice, a great determination. Despite my concern for Bob and my own skepticism that he might have difficultly succeeding with this plan, it was a very uplifting moment, and one I will not soon forget. We shook hands and Bob limped slowly out of the office. As time passed, I put that day out of my thoughts and returned to business as usual. One day, about six months later, I was back in the office and saw a new patient casually walking down the hallway being escorted by the nurse. Once he was put into a room, I grabbed his medical chart, walked into the room and introduced by self as Dr. Moyad. As we shook hands, he looked at me and said "I told you I would be back doc." I must admit, I was a bit bewildered. I had never seen this person before, but something was strangely familiar about him. We stared at each other awkwardly for a moment, and I said to him "What can I do for you today sir." He looked at me again with a grin on his face and said "Nothing, I'm fine." Again, I felt a strange feeling of familiarity with this person, but for the life of me, I could not recall where I may have seen him before. I quickly searched my thoughts......maybe I've seen him at the grocery store or at the fitness club or perhaps at a party. After a few seconds, I gave up and said to the patient, "I just need to take a quick look through your medical chart." He nodded his head in agreement and I looked down at his medical file and opened the chart. I started to get goose bumps when I realized who he was. It was Bob! Except for his eyes and his voice he was a completely different man. The first thing I did was to admit that I had no idea who he was until I looked down at the chart and recognized his name from the previous visit. We *both had a good laugh and I asked him how in the world he lost all of that weight, especially since he had trouble walking down the hallway the last time I saw him. Bob told me that he just **stuck to the plan and was determined to change his life**. Not only did he achieve the weight loss goal that we had set, but his achievements far surpassed my expectations. He lost enough weight to bring his body mass from a morbid condition to one that was near ideal for his body height. I told Bob that he had done more than his fair share of the bargain and if he still had significant pain or disability, I would be happy to offer him surgery. He looked at me and said "No thanks, doc. I feel better now than I have in many, many years." When I asked him how much pain and disability he was having from his joints he said it was minimal now compared to almost a 10 out 10 just six months earlier. We spent some more time chatting and he left that day. I never saw Bob again after that.*

Clearly this kind of change does not happen every day and in certain cases the challenges faced by some disabled patients are too significant to completely overcome without medical intervention. Furthermore, it's atypical to see a patient with severe joint destruction go from the worst kind of pain to having almost a normal life through weight loss alone. But every now and then, amazing things do happen, and Bob's story is just one of these examples. The real take home message behind this story is how this individual overcame incredible odds and achieved an enormous improvement in his health and well-being: He simply stuck to the plan and was determined to succeed.

So why is it so hard for people with chronic illness and disability to eat less? One explanation is that it's often quite hard for the body and mind to accept change. We can become so accustomed to a particular pattern or behavior that the routine is ingrained in our bodies and in our minds. In essence our mind is on "autopilot" and we act and respond almost unconsciously. Those with disabilities, therefore, must become conscious again of these eating patterns and realize it can take a significant amount of time for our physiologic set point for hunger to change.

The first step we need to take in order to control overconsumption is to accept that we must significantly reduce our calories in order to realign our daily consumption with our actual nutritional needs.

The next step is to reprogram how we think, and to use positive thoughts to help us achieve our goals. Negative thoughts will work against us. For example:

"I need to starve myself." But starving yourself will lead to a serious deterioration in your health or possibly death. Now why would you ever commit yourself to do such a thing in an attempt to become healthier? You obviously would not. Rather, your internal monologue should sound more like this: "I am determined to realign my consumption to fit the actual needs of my body, so that I will become a healthier person." In other words, keep your thoughts positive!

Lastly, all the recommendations and techniques presented in the diet section of this program must be applied with the same determination, perhaps more, in those with disability. For instance, we know that anxiety and stress can lead to overconsumption by reducing our sense of control. In this situation, eating is a maladaptive attempt to seek comfort. However, eating will not satisfy this void and, in fact, it may complicate anxiety and depression further.

Those with physical challenges and disabilities are prone to anxiety and stress, especially if they lack the correct coping methods and adequate social network. In this case, we can rely on our methods of stress reduction to change our behavior, improve our diet and better our health.

Exercise and physical activity must also be modified when disease or physical impairment occurs. Notice that I say we must modify certain activities. This certainly does not mean that we abandon all activities or stop trying to exercise altogether. In fact, exercise is crucial to one's health in this circumstance.

Although disability is an accepted medical term, some in the lay community incorrectly equate this with the term "inability." This is far from the truth, as many people with disabilities will tell you that they are quite capable of doing numerous activities just as well, or even better, than those without disability. Nevertheless, we must appreciate and acknowledge the fact that certain activities may be more challenging or even painful for some disabled individuals. But some form of exercise is imperative to improve health and wellness.

Let's consider the example of someone with paraplegia (a partial or complete loss of function in two limbs, usually the legs). Certainly, there are activities which simply cannot be accomplished. However, there are many exercises and activities involving the upper limbs and torso which are critical for weight maintenance, musculoskeletal stamina, cardiovascular fitness, stress reduction and other health benefits. For patients like Bob, who are afflicted with severe joint arthritis, walking distance and speed are often considerably reduced. However, it is usually possible to take short walks on flat ground with proper orthotics.

In addition, there are several excellent low impact options that can help improve muscle tone and fitness. For instance, certain elliptical exercise machines that effectively reduce forces on the lower body may be a good choice. Pool exercises are another activity choice, as the forces across a given joint or limb are decreased in water. What may be considered to be mild exercise in those without injury or physical impairment can have enormous benefits in people who are afflicted with disabilities.

Furthermore, the increased health achieved by a so called "small or modest" gain in exercise is exponentially higher in those with significant disability in comparison to an elite athlete. For example, a long distance runner who normally runs 7 miles per day would gain little from increasing his or her workout to 8 miles per day, in terms of his or her health. It fact, it could even have a negative consequence in the form of an overuse injury, which is not uncommon in elite athletes.

Now take the case of someone who has recently lost the ability to walk. This person can choose to approach the situation in one of two ways: He or she may decide that since they are quite limited now, exercise is of little value and neglect this component of life, which would be a terrible mistake. The other scenario is for this person to realize that being sedentary is very detrimental to one's physical and mental health. Therefore, every little bit of activity and exercise that he or she can comfortably perform, no matter how seemingly small, can actually have huge benefits on cardiovascular, musculoskeletal and mental health.

Combined with the proper diet, a routine exercise regimen will allow those with disabilities and physical challenges to significantly increase their level of health.

ADAPTING TO CHANGE:

Evolution is another important concept for us to grasp when considering our health and wellness. In the Healthy 4 program, the concept of evolution has to do with the idea that health as well as life is in constant flux. Because of this constant change, we are never exactly the same person at any two given points in time.

Some changes are a normal part of the aging process, while others may be due to an illness or injury. Some of the more difficult changes to accept can cause us to fixate on what has been lost. On the one hand, a certain amount of grief is not only understandable but is also healthy from the perspective that it is a normal coping mechanism that allows us to put the past behind us.

On the other hand, prolonged periods of grief, sadness or regret prevent us from moving forward and can cause mental anguish and stress that further diminishes our health, both mentally and physically. Overcoming challenges and adapting to change is a process that involves letting go of our grief and appreciating what we have at the present time.

The stages of grief have been described previously by *Dr. Elisabeth Kubler-Ross* and can be thought of as evolutionary process as well. The stages have been said to occur in the following order:

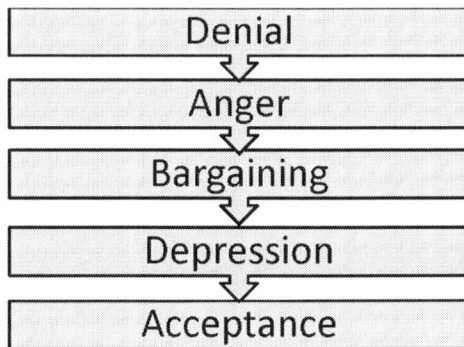

Denial
Anger
Bargaining
Depression
Acceptance

Although not every person progresses through each of these stages or follows this exact pattern, it does serve as a useful model of the adaptation process that can occur during a significant loss or life changing event. Notice that the last stage is acceptance, which we absolutely must enter in order to adapt to change and thrive.

When significant loss occurs, such as a substantial injury or disability, it is critical to accept this change as an inevitable part of life. The length of time that it takes to adapt to change obviously depends on the significance of the event and the individual's own nature and ability. We can all improve our own ability to adapt to change by using the techniques and applying the concepts that will be discussed in the next two sections on stress reduction and spirituality.

For now, realize that evolution is inevitable and that every change, both good and bad, is a natural part of life. Moreover, we all experience periods of life where our health deteriorates and improves. The key to unlocking our full potential is to make the most of our health at the present time. We all have the ability to become healthier and happier today, no matter what our circumstance.

CHAPTER NINE:
BUILDING AN EXERCISE ROUTINE

We all know physical activity and exercise is important for each one of us and that combined with the appropriate diet, it can significantly improve our health and well-being. There are many different types of exercises that can be performed. We will cover a variety of them and their health benefits.

Before we dive into the specifics, remember that we are trying to assemble several key components of health into a practical program that all of us can use daily. Thus, we started with diet and we proposed that you begin your process in a stepwise progression. Recall the early stages of our diet program summary:

DAY 1-15:

➤ Record your daily calorie intake in your diet log

DAY 16-30:

➤ Set a calorie consumption goal and begin to modify calorie intake based on this goal

➤ Begin your new exercise regimen

Notice that we do not incorporate the exercise routine in the first period from day 1-15. There are several good reasons for this.

First, to avoid being overwhelmed with too many new tasks, we build up the Healthy 4 program in a stepwise manner. Next, you need to focus on accurately recording your normal calorie consumption pattern in the first stage, so that we can build upon this knowledge in later stages of the program. Last and most important of all, adding a new exercise routine during the early stage can alter your normal pattern of consumption, which would prevent us from accurately assessing your routine daily calorie intake.

For instance, an increase in exercise can lead to an increase in calories. During this first 15 days, the goal is to discover approximately how many calories you routinely consume and compare this to what is considered standard and most beneficial to a person of similar size and age. This will give you valuable information for the future and help you determine if you need to start restricting calories and, if so, by how much.

If you have a particular exercise regimen already, by all means you should continue it. The main point during the first 15 days is to do everything you normally do for diet and exercise.

In some situations, you may even decide that you prefer your own exercise plan instead, and wish to continue with your own routine. This might be the case if you are very active and have already developed an advanced workout routine. In other cases, you may have an injury or disability that precludes you from doing some of the exercises in this plan.

In any case, our objective is to encourage you to participate in an active exercise program that is both fun and sustainable for you. This will allow you to consistently incorporate exercise with your other Healthy 4 components to maximize your health potential.

TYPES OF EXERCISE:

Generally speaking we can describe our exercises in terms of cardiovascular health and musculoskeletal health. We also can categorize exercise into aerobic (oxygen requiring) and anaerobic (non-oxygen requiring) activities. Aerobic or cardiovascular conditioning often involves those activities that require more endurance and a prolonged increase in heart beat. While anaerobic or musculoskeletal conditioning often involves short bursts of exercise that involve less endurance and more power.

<u>Example of Cardiovascular (Aerobic) Activity</u>:

- ✓ Jogging
- ✓ Elliptical machine
- ✓ Swimming
- ✓ Jumping rope
- ✓ Biking
- ✓ Dancing

<u>Examples of Musculoskeletal Strengthening (Anaerobic) Activity</u>:

- ✓ Lifting weights
- ✓ Short sprints
- ✓ High jump

Incidentally, the use of the word anaerobic (without oxygen) does not mean than we do not require oxygen during these activities. Rather it refers to the ability of our cells to burn sugar without the immediate use of oxygen. In reality, most common exercises are a mixture of both anaerobic and aerobic type of training. Just realize that some exercises focus more on the health of your heart and circulatory system while others are more important for our bones, muscles and connective tissues.

We will begin with specific exercises that strengthen our muscles and connective tissues. Some may ask why this type of exercise is so important or why we are not focusing on activities that typically make us sweat. One of the main reasons that resistance training or musculoskeletal training is important is because it adds bone density and reduces the rate of bone loss during our lifetime.

Significant bone density loss is a serious and common problem as we age. Often referred to as osteopenia or osteoporosis, this condition can lead to major fractures and is a common cause of sickness and death in the elderly. Starting at about 25 - 30 years of age, human beings begin to lose bone mass at a steady rate for the rest of their lives. Resistance exercise will aid in building bone mass and ultimately preserve more bone density as we get older.

Furthermore, our bones are connected to one another through different types of joints. Many of these joints incur tremendous stresses throughout our lifetime that can lead to joint damage and arthritis. Certain exercises specifically build muscle density and strengthen ligaments and tendons that serve to protect our joints.

Another important benefit of resistance training and building lean muscle mass is that it increases the body's metabolism. This allows us to burn more calories throughout the day, even when we are sedentary. The key to this type of training, however, is to perform all exercises with good technique, paying particular attention to posture at all times. Done incorrectly, all exercises can be counterproductive and, worse, cause injury that could potentially damage our health rather than improve it.

Before we discuss specific exercises and routines, it is important for you to realize that we all have different experience levels. Some of you may be very familiar with the exercises listed in this book. If this is the case, please read through them anyway, as you may be able to pick up a few pointers along the way. Others may have limited experience and may benefit from hiring a qualified trainer to ensure that these exercises are performed safely and properly.

Don't worry if you can't do all the exercises listed. No matter what your previous level of physical condition, there are several activities and exercises that you can incorporate into your life to improve your fitness. For those of you new to exercise or with health concerns, we recommend consulting with your physician before engaging in an exercise routine.

A variety of exercise pictures containing instructions can also be found on the Healthy4.com website for your review. Let's begin with some common muscle strengthening and resistance exercises.

SIT UPS:

These core strengthening exercises are very important for correct posture and help to relieve the stresses on your low back and lumbar spine.

➢ To begin, lay on the floor with your back against a flat padded surface with the knees bent

➢ Next fold your arms across your chest – not behind your neck – and slowly lift your back, neck and head off the ground as a single unit

➢ Avoid touching your chin against your chest during this maneuver. Additionally avoid placing your hands behind your head. This creates the tendency to push your head forward which will place strain on your neck

➢ With your feet planted on the ground, lift your back, neck and head several inches off the floor as a single unit. Concentrate on contracting your stomach muscles throughout this exercise

You will often see people in the gym who try to raise their back all the way off the ground until their chest touches their knees. This often places increased stress on your spine which could lead to injury. The proper way to perform a sit up is to keep your feet firmly on the ground with your knees bent. Alternatively, you can rest your legs over a bench keeping a 90 degree bend at the hips and knees. The goal is to elevate your torso/upper body several inches off the ground while focusing on your stomach muscles.

You should feel muscle contraction primarily in your abdomen and no place else. Again, avoid lifting your back too high off the ground or curling your neck into a c-shape. Your back and neck should remain straight when performing this exercise. It helps to point your eyes straight upward during the exercise, rather than trying to look forward by flexing your neck, which puts added pressure on your cervical spine.

➢ I recommend that beginners perform 2-3 sets of these exercises three times per week

WHAT'S THE DIFFERENCE BETWEEN REPETITIONS AND SETS?

Note: A **repetition** is a single maneuver or movement of a particular exercise. A **set** describes the number of repetitions performed in a row. For example, if you perform 10 sit ups in a row, than you have performed 10 repetitions during that exercise set.

NEVER FOCUS ON THE NUMBER OF REPETITIONS!

The reason you should never focus on the number of repetitions of an exercise is because it is absolutely meaningless! As you know we all have different abilities and strengths. For example, let's say I tell you to perform 15 sit ups in a row (15 repetitions per set.) If one person is actually able to perform 50 sit ups, then he or she would not be training hard enough and so it is of no value.

On the other hand, if another person is able to perform only 5 perfectly executed sit ups, one of two things happen. The first is that the person becomes frustrated because he or she is unable to achieve 15 repetitions. This frustration will eventually be overwhelming and the person will quit. Remember, exercise should be fun as well as attainable, so let's avoid feelings of frustration.

The second thing that often happens is that the individual starts to concentrate on this meaningless number of repetitions during the exercise and he or she loses focus on proper technique. In this case, the repetitions become sloppy, counterproductive and possibly even dangerous.

To look at it another way, it doesn't matter if your muscle becomes fatigued at 5 sit ups or 50 sit ups, so long as they are done properly. What matters is that correct form is used throughout the movement and you concentrate on the target muscle group in the actual exercise. It's often best to continue to do the exercise until your muscle becomes fatigued. That is, you should stop the exercise once you feel that you are no longer able to continue without cheating or altering your proper form. We urge against exercising beyond your abilities. Fatigue is not the same as pain and if you begin to feel pain or cramping, all activity should stop.

To revisit our last example, if you fatigue at 5 correctly performed sit ups, you will be training your own body as optimally as someone who can do 50 sit ups (not to mention, your work outs will be much quicker). Nevertheless, muscle fibers do tend to adapt quickly, and soon the number of repetitions that you will be able to safely perform will increase.

So how many sets of a particular exercise should one perform during a daily workout? Well, that is a little more difficult to say. There is no exact number that I can give, because that depends on several factors. Keep in mind that sets, like repetitions, can encourage poor form if arbitrarily determined.

It is more important to monitor how you feel during and after a workout to gauge if you are doing the right number of sets. There is a fine line between feeling sore after a workout and feeling good after a workout. If you are constantly sore after workouts or prior to starting your next workout, then it's likely that you are overtraining. Remember, pain is our enemy here.

However, to standardize your workout, I will make the following suggestions: For beginners, I recommend doing no more than 3 sets of resistance exercises per workout for every major muscle group that you train. For example, if you are trying to target your chest, doing 3 sets total during that day's workout should be more than sufficient. With time, you may find that you can comfortably increase the number of sets. Regarding the number of repetitions however, again I would recommend that you focus primarily on properly exercising your muscle, rather than performing a certain number.

PUSH UPS:

Push ups are an excellent way to strengthen your chest and arms, especially if you do not have time to visit a gym or you do not have access to a club.

> ➤ Begin with your arms shoulder width apart and your eyes pointed forward
> ➤ Keep your entire body as level to the floor as possible during this exercise. Your buttock should not be higher than your back
> ➤ Lower your entire body slowly in a controlled fashion until your chest barely touches the floor
> ➤ Next, immediately raise your body, again keeping as level as possible with your eyes pointed forward

It is important that this exercise be performed in a controlled, continual manner.

Avoid prolonged rest by locking your elbows straight at the top of the exercise or resting your chest at the bottom of the movement. Remember that proper technique, not the number of repetitions, is what matters. The goal is to tire your muscle out using perfect form. If performing a few correct pushups seems too difficult, especially at the beginner level, an alternate way is to rest your knees and legs on the floor and push just your torso and upper body off the floor.

➢ I recommend 3 sets of pushups 2 times per week

BENCH PRESS:

Like the push up, this exercise is an excellent way to strengthen your chest and arms. This can be performed using free weights or by using closed circuit training equipment. Free weights demand that you also control the proper direction of the movement in addition to performing the work required to move the object. Free weights and machines are both very good methods of resistance training, although free weights are perhaps a bit more difficult to master if you are not familiar with using them. The key again is to use proper technique to avoid injury or over use.

If you prefer free weights, you should use a safety spotter who can assist you during this exercise in case you can't return the weight to its resting position or you need to suddenly stop the movement. The actual applied technique will be similar, whether you prefer to use circuit machines or free weights.

➢ Slowly lower the weight towards the chest in the case of free weights or slowly raise the weight in the case of most bench press machines
➢ Keep your feet firmly planted and your buttock, back and head resting flat against the bench throughout the entire exercise. Cheating by lifting your buttock or arching your low back during this movement decreases its effectiveness and can lead to injury
➢ Similar to the push up, the bench press should be well controlled and constant. Avoid resting the weight on your chest or locking your elbows straight at the top of the movement, which disrupts the fluidity of the movement
➢ Avoid heavy weights or heavy lifting. The objective, like always, is to feel a healthy fatigue but NEVER pain!

The idea of "no pain no gain" may seem useful to certain professional athletes who make a living from their respective sport, but it is not beneficial for healthy living and longevity. In fact, this philosophy will more likely lead to injury and a reduction in your overall well-being, rather than promote health. This does not mean that you should never break a sweat or exercise without vigor. Our bodies are resilient and need to be pushed at times to allow them to adapt and improve. However, if a particular movement hurts, something is probably wrong. I cannot stress enough that the best way to prevent injury is to adhere to proper technique and concentrate on the actual muscle group that is being trained. Forget about trying to see how much weight you can lift or the number of repetitions that you can perform.

➢ I recommend 3 sets of bench presses 2 times per week
➢ Alternatively you can combine both bench press and push ups for a total of 3 sets 2 times per week

PULL UPS OR PULL DOWNS:

These basic exercises target the major muscle groups of the upper back. A pull up is done with a sturdy overhanging bar that can support the weight of your body. These can be done at home or in the gym. Affordable bars can be purchased online or at a sporting goods store. Pull downs do require the use of a fitness center or gym, although they can also be performed at home with store bought exercise equipment. Again, the basic movements are similar and the choice depends on your preference, ability level and access to equipment.

To begin a proper pull up:

➢ Keep your arms more than shoulder width apart and grab the bar over handed with your palms facing away from you
➢ Slowly pull your body upward until your chin is at the level of your hands
➢ Lower yourself in a similar slow and controlled manner
➢ Pull ups can be difficult depending on your body weight and experience. If you have trouble with lifting all your weight, there are machines at many gyms that effectively reduce your body weight, thus making the movement easier. Either way, avoid jerky movements and focus on contracting your upper back muscles when performing this exercise

Alternatively, you can perform a pull down in a similar manner:

- ➤ Begin this exercise in a seated position, again with your arms more than shoulder width apart
- ➤ Grab the bar in an over handed position and slowly pull the bar down until it gently touches your upper chest
- ➤ Next, slowly allow the bar to ascend while providing some resistance to ensure that you are continually working your muscles throughout the entire exercise
- ➤ Your back, neck and head should always be in a straight line and your body should remain in a relatively stationary position. Only your arms should be moving during this activity. Thus, you are raising and lowering the bar through your upper limbs, while concentrating on contracting your back muscles during the entire movement. You should feel your upper back muscles doing most of the work rather than your arms
- ➤ Begin with 2-3 sets of pull ups, pull downs or both 2 times per week

SQUATS:

These exercises are excellent for strengthening your core lower body muscles: including your gluteus (buttock) and quadriceps and hamstring (thigh) muscles. You can do these at home or at the gym with added resistance. Let's review the technique of the basic squat:

- ➤ Stand with your legs planted shoulder width apart and place a chair or bench behind you to ensure that you do not squat too deeply which puts unnecessary stress on your knee joints
- ➤ Begin by slowly lowering yourself until your buttock makes contact with the seat or bench behind you. Your knees should be at approximately a 45 to 60 degree angle at this point (your knees should never bend beyond 90 degrees)
- ➤ Next, slowly raise yourself upwards keeping your eyes forward until you are standing almost straight and repeat the process

Never bend your knees beyond a 90 degrees angle during this exercise. Bending 45 to 60 degrees is still very effective while putting less strain on the lower back, hips and knees. If you prefer to do these at the gym, you can add weight to your routine. However, as previously stated, always use excellent technique and focus more on the quality of the movement rather than amount of weight used or number of repetitions performed.

> ➤ Again, I would recommend starting off with 2-3 sets of squats 2 times per week

There are many other types of resistance activities and variations that you may encounter in your training. Although you will undoubtedly add different exercises and vary your routine over time, the core exercises described here will provide the foundation for anyone attempting to improve their musculoskeletal fitness.

There is one final point to be made about beginning these exercises. At the start, I suggest that you target one specific muscle group at one time, rather than performing so called "circuit training" in which you move back and forth between different muscle groups. An example of circuit training would be to perform a set of sits ups, push-ups and squats, one right after another. Although this type of training can also be effective, it is generally easier to gauge your muscle fatigue by concentrating on a single muscle group before moving on to the next.

Let's move on to a discussion about cardiovascular training, which helps lower the risk of many preventable diseases including high blood pressure, obesity, diabetes, peripheral vascular disease, stroke and heart disease. The combination of strength training and cardiovascular training most efficiently boosts your metabolism, allowing you to optimally burn food calories and maximizes your overall health.

Cardiovascular activities increase your heart rate. The ones I list here serve not only to protect your heart, but tend to cause less stress on your joints, potentially improving both cardiovascular and musculoskeletal fitness.

Knowing just how much to increase your heart rate is an essential part of beginning a cardiovascular routine. **Target heart rates** have been established to help guide your workout effort. The target heart rate is based on your age and is a percentage of your maximum heart rate (defined as the fastest your heart beats under normal exercise conditions.) Most often, exercise charts use between 60 and 80 percent of your **maximum heart rate** to establish an appropriate target or goal.

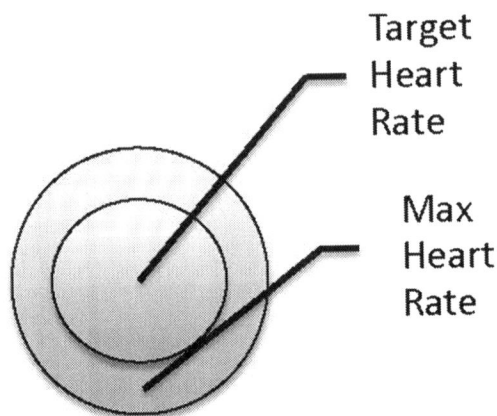

For instance, let's say an individual's maximum heart rate based on their age is 200 beats per minute. Using the 60 and 80 percent range, their target rate would fall between 120 and 160 beats per minute. Obviously, the higher up this range, the harder your heart will work.

As we have stated in previous sections, I don't want you to get caught up in the numbers. If you are unable to maintain your target heart rate throughout your entire work out, it is not the end of the world. Any sustained activity or exercise that allows the heart to pump faster than it does when sedentary is good for your health and should be incorporated into your daily life. However, as we come closer to achieving the target heart rate, exercise efficiency increases, which is beneficial to our health and well-being. If you have any health concerns, ask your doctor before starting an exercise program.

To find out what your target heart rate should be based on your age, you can ask to see these charts at your local fitness center or go to our website at www. healthy4.com.

ELLIPTICAL MACHINE:

Although this requires that you belong to a gym or purchase your own equipment, the elliptical machine is one of the best types of exercises to increase your heart rate while providing a low amount of impact to your joints. I have recommended this type of exercise to most of my patients with lower extremity joint diseases such as rheumatoid arthritis or osteoarthritis.

In case you have not seen or used this equipment before, it basically is a standing machine that has two foot pedals connected to a pivot arm. Its name is derived from the type of motion that is produced with your legs as you exercise. Rather than a stationary bicycle which allows more circular motion in a seated position, this machine allows more of an elliptical motion in an erect position.

Some of these machines are equipped with sensor monitors to allow you track your heart rate during this exercise. Whether you use a digital monitor or do it the old fashion way by checking your own pulse rate, it is important to know how hard your heart is working.

SWIMMING AND WATER AEROBICS:

These exercises significantly reduce the forces placed on your joints due to the buoyancy effect of water. The reason that I favor this type of exercise is that it can be a great cardiovascular exercise for just about anyone, from an Olympic Athlete to an elderly person who may have discomfort during weight bearing exercise.

Many fitness centers offer water aerobics. If membership cost is a factor, there may be discount memberships at local recreation clubs such as the YMCA. In addition, many communities offer open pool hours throughout the school year or water aerobics training during certain periods at reduced rates.

Proper swim gear is an important consideration as it adds to your comfort level. You should purchase a set of swimming goggles and nose or ear plugs as well, which will help you avoid any irritation to your mucous membranes from chlorination. Being relaxed in the water will improve your chance of maintaining this activity over the long haul.

STATIONARY AND ROAD BICYCLE:

Whether you enjoy the stationary bike or you prefer to get outside and do some road work, bike riding is a very good exercise which also tends to be less stressful on your joints compared to running. Remember to wear a protective helmet if biking outside. Although our bodies can be very resilient, a seemingly benign or low speed accident can have devastating consequences if we are misfortunate enough to fall in the wrong way. A helmet is an easy way to reduce your risk and protect your life.

Occasionally, people who do a lot of biking or who have knee problems complain of knee discomfort. For people with a history of knee injuries or arthritis, raising the seat level higher will decrease the stress on your knee cap. Raising the seat reduces the amount of knee joint flexion and as a result it reduces the amount of stress on the front of your knee. This can often improve your comfort level. Remember, however, if you feel pain when performing a particular exercise, its best to stop and talk with your doctor before resuming bicycling or other aerobic activity.

WALKING:

You don't always have to get your heart rate up to 160 beats per minute or sweat profusely to improve your health. If time is limited try walking up the stairs instead of taking the elevator. If you enjoy golfing, leave the electric cart behind and walk the course if you can. Taking a half hour walk a day by yourself or with your family is a great way to promote health and well-being.

You should purchase comfortable walking shoes with adequate shock absorption. Bare feet or slippers may feel fine to you, but shoes with good arch support and shock absorption are more forgiving on the other joints of your body such as the ankles, knees and lower back.

RUNNING VS LOW IMPACT EXERCISE:

A review of exercise would not be complete if I were to neglect all the runners out there. Jogging certainly is an excellent way to burn calories and improve your cardiac fitness. Some runners may not agree with what I am about to say, nevertheless, I do have some concerns about certain high impact running activity. In my experience as an Orthopedic Surgeon, I've seen two different demographics of patients. Those who are older with normal "wear and tear" joint problems and younger, active individuals with overuse injuries and early arthritis. Many of the latter are passionate runners and participate in high impact activities.

I will be the first to admit that we do not have good scientific evidence that proves that exercise such as long distance running will lead to problems down the road; however, I have seen enough patients over the years to take pause. I would not go so far as to say that all avid runners should avoid the exercise that they love, especially since it is good for the heart and helps maintain optimal weight. Rather my message is this: If you are seeking to improve your health, any of the exercises that have been described here will help you achieve that goal. Running is not necessary to achieve excellent cardiovascular and musculoskeletal fitness.

If you are a runner and enjoy this form of fitness, just remember one of the basic tenants in life: MODERATION IS KEY! I do not mean to single out any one particular group because this philosophy is important for all people, not just runners. However, I do find that avid runners seem to have a higher percentage of individuals who are obsessive about their routine and sometimes over-train to the point of injury. Healthy living involves a balanced lifestyle.

So how do we determine how much exercise is too much? Unfortunately, there is no easy answer, since it depends on many factors such as the type and duration of the exercise, one's age, prior conditioning and our unique physiologic reserves. However, here are some important rules to follow when incorporating an exercise routine into your life:

➤ Never exercise through pain or significant discomfort
➤ Eat a well-balanced diet with approximately 30% of your calories or more from high quality protein such as chicken, fish, egg whites or dairy products
➤ Get plenty of sleep; at least 7 to 8 hours per night if possible
➤ Watch for common signs and symptoms of overtraining: joint or limb pain, chronic fatigue, swelling, increased frequency of illness such as the common cold or frequent cold sores, excessive muscle soreness or

prolonged recuperation time between work outs, loss of interest or motivation for exercise

➤ Listen to your body first. If something seems wrong or unsafe, follow your instinct rather than listening to another person, especially at the start of an exercise program. With time and experience most people become more in tune with their limitations. Sometimes clichés are fitting: Better to be safe than sorry

➤ Set realistic goals that promote consistency and longevity, rather than focusing on short term, sporadic objectives (such as the need to fit into a swim suit by summer). Remember, Rome was not built in a day!

➤ Exercise should be fun. Find ways to vary your routine to keep yourself interested and to prevent your body from reaching a plateau with a particular routine. Sometimes finding a workout buddy or partner can be very helpful as well

➤ Always warm up at the beginning of any exercise routine to allow proper blood flow to your muscles and connective tissues. Spend at least 5-10 minutes on stretching exercises before ramping up your activity level to decrease the risk of injury

The cardiovascular exercises listed should be incorporated into a consistent routine. **30 minutes at least 3 times a week** is a good goal to pursue and will significantly boost your health and fitness. Remember to find out what your target heart rate should be and try to achieve this whenever possible during your exercise routine. If you are unable to do this or have limited time, try to increase your daily activity and movement by walking more often, for example. Just by putting down the remote control or getting out of your chair a few more times a day can help you to improve your health and well-being and prepare your body for more vigorous activity.

Remember exercise, like diet, is a way of life and may require reprioritizing some of your goals. Without your health, it is difficult to enjoy any pursuit in this world. Since proper exercise and diet are two of the most basic and efficient means of becoming healthier, we should all strive to spend a reasonable amount of time and effort on improving these aspects of our life.

So now that we have discussed several different types of musculoskeletal and cardiovascular exercises in detail, let's put it all together and form a few typical routines that you may use in your daily practice. Keep in mind that these are suggested routines and serve as good starting points. However, there are no hard and fast rules to follow here. Depending on your current activity level, experience and abilities, you may want to modify these routines. Over time, we all need to vary our exercise regimen somewhat to keep them interesting and fresh. But for now, these routines will serve as an excellent starting point for most.

I have provided three basic exercise routines that have been categorized into beginner, intermediate and advanced. Although these are somewhat arbitrarily designed, they do provide a solid framework for us to utilize during our exercise program. Some of you may be able to jump right to the advanced level or beyond due to a high degree of fitness and experience. Others may be just getting back into exercise and find that the beginner routine is more than enough.

Regardless of your current activity level, it is important to be honest with yourself and choose an exercise program that is right for you. The best health gains come from consistency rather than occasional or sporadic activity. Therefore, feel free to modify your routine if it allows you to stick to the program. Either way, make it a frequent and regular part of your life. You will be glad that you did, I promise you!

<u>Level One – Beginner</u>:

This may be appropriate for someone who has been inconsistent or has had a significant hiatus from exercise. It may also be useful for someone who is not very familiar with these types of activities and is looking for a change in their workout.

<u>Day 1</u>:

- ✓ Cardio training: **30 minutes** elliptical machine, swimming, stationary bike or equivalent
- ✓ Core resistance training: push ups and/or bench press **2 sets**
- ✓ Core resistance training: pull ups and/or pull downs **2 sets**
- ✓ Sit ups: **2 sets**

Day 2: Rest

Day 3:

- ✓ Cardio training: **30 minutes** elliptical machine, swimming, stationary bike or equivalent
- ✓ Core resistance training: squats **2 sets**
- ✓ Sit ups: **2 sets**

Day 4: Rest

Day 5:

- ✓ Cardio training: **30 minutes** elliptical machine, swimming, stationary bike or equivalent
- ✓ Core resistance training: push ups and/or bench press **2 sets**
- ✓ Core resistance training: pull ups and/or pull downs **2 sets**
- ✓ Sit ups: **2 sets**

Day 6 & 7: Rest then Repeat

This is a 7 day cycle that repeats after day 7. This workout allows adequate time for the beginner to recuperate and minimize this risk of over training. Note: these rest days are necessary for recovery; however one can continue to find ways to remain active on non workout days. For example, taking a walk or using the stairs at work are good ways to boost your metabolism and should be sought out every day.

Level Two – Intermediate:

Day I:

- ✓ Cardio training: **30 minutes** elliptical machine, swimming, stationary bike or equivalent
- ✓ Core resistance training: push ups and/or bench press **3 sets**

✓ Core resistance training: pull ups and/or pull downs **3 sets**
✓ Sit ups: **2-3 sets**

Day 2: Rest

Day 3:

✓ Cardio training: **30 minutes** elliptical machine, swimming, stationary bike or equivalent
✓ Core resistance training: squats **2-3 sets**
✓ Sit ups: **2-3 sets**

Day 4: Rest

Day 5:

✓ Cardio training: **30 minutes** elliptical machine, swimming, stationary bike or equivalent
✓ Core resistance training: push ups and/or bench press **3 sets**
✓ Core resistance training: pull ups and/or pull downs **3 sets**
✓ Sit ups: **2-3 sets**

Day 6: Rest

Day 7: Rest or Repeat

This program is similar to the beginner level except for small increases in the musculoskeletal portions of the regimen. In addition, on day 7 of this program the individual has the option to take another day off if fatigue is present. If energy levels are fine, the individual also has the option to repeat the cycle one day earlier, essentially making it a 6 day workout program.

Level Three – Advanced:

Day 1:

- ✓ Cardio training: **30 minutes** elliptical machine, swimming, stationary bike or equivalent
- ✓ Core resistance training: push ups and/or bench press: **4 sets**
- ✓ Core resistance training: pull ups and/or pull downs: **4 sets**

Day 2:

- ✓ Cardio training: **30 minutes** elliptical machine, swimming, stationary bike or equivalent
- ✓ Core resistance training: squats: **3 sets**
- ✓ Sit ups: **3 sets**

Day 3: Rest

Day 4:

- ✓ Cardio training: **30 minutes** elliptical machine, swimming, stationary bike or equivalent
- ✓ Core resistance training: push ups and/or bench press: **4 sets**
- ✓ Core resistance training: pull ups and/or pull downs: **4 sets**

Day 5:

- ✓ Cardio training: **30 minutes** elliptical machine, swimming, stationary bike or equivalent
- ✓ Core resistance training: squats: **3 sets**
- ✓ Sit ups: **3 sets**

Day 6: Rest

Day 7: Rest or Repeat

Remember the exercise programs provided are suggested routines that are meant to provide an efficient and balanced fitness routine for most people. You may need to modify them somewhat depending on your abilities and level of fatigue. With experience you will find other exercises that work well for you, too.

This program can be approached in a step wise progression starting from beginner, then working your way to advanced for those of you new to an exercise routine. The time to progress from one level to the next depends on your comfort level. Importantly, all three of these programs require only a few hours per week and will yield good results if you adhere to them, along with a proper diet.

Thus far, we have discussed diet and exercise, two of the four major components of health. Individually each has the ability to improve your fitness. However, combining both programs into a single regimen and making this part of your daily life will significantly improve your health.

In summary, the diet and exercise components of our program are as follows:

HEALTHY 4 SUMMARY PLAN FOR DIET AND EXERCISE:

DAY 1 – DAY 15:

❖ Diet: Begin recording your daily calorie consumption each day for the first 15 days (review nutrition labels)

❖ Exercise Program: None (continue with your normal activity and exercise routines until stage two of the program)

DAY 16 – DAY 30:

❖ Diet: Continue recording your daily calorie consumption

❖ Diet: Use the information from your calorie consumption log to establish a daily calorie consumption limit (such as 2000 calories)

❖ Diet: Use the following dieting pearls to assist you:
   ✓ Avoid eating until full
   ✓ Eat small portions or reduce your meal size
   ✓ Eat <u>more</u> frequently during the day versus one or two large meals
   ✓ Don't wait until your hunger is strong before you eat
   ✓ SLOW DOWN when you eat
   ✓ Pack your own food and carry nutritional supplements with you
   ✓ Avoid eating as a reflex to hunger (assess for abnormal cues)
   ✓ Avoid buffets and all you can eat menus
   ✓ Consume low calorie foods and drinks
   ✓ Count your calories and set daily goals
   ✓ Keep yourself well hydrated
   ✓ Drink water rather high calorie drinks
   ✓ Try a healthy snack <u>before</u> a meal

✓ Forget about adhering to traditional course meals (i.e. 3 or 4 courses)

✓ DON'T feel the need to clear your plate and STOP eating once you meet your dietary goals

✓ Never eat before going to sleep

✓ Associate positive thought to healthy foods

✓ Eat a well-balanced diet

✓ Consume most of your fats from **un**saturated, **non**-trans fat sources

✓ Don't prepare or cover your food with unhealthy toppings

❖ Exercise Program: Start beginner level one program (or higher depending on comfort and experience)

DAY 1 (DAY 16 OVERALL):
Cardio training: **30 minutes** elliptical machine, swimming, stationary bike or equivalent
Core resistance training: push ups and/or bench press **2 sets**
Core resistance training: pull ups and/or pull downs **2 sets**
Sit ups: **2 sets**

DAY 2 (DAY 17 OVERALL): Rest

DAY 3 (DAY 18 OVERALL):
Cardio training: **30 minutes** elliptical machine, swimming, stationary bike or equivalent
Core resistance training: squats **2 sets**
Sit ups: **2 sets**

DAY 4 (DAY 19 OVERALL): REST

DAY 5 (DAY 20 OVERALL):
Cardio training: **30 minutes**
Core resistance training: push ups and/or bench press **2 sets**

Core resistance training: pull ups and/or pull downs **2 sets**

Sit ups **2 sets**

DAY 6 & 7 (DAY 21 & 22 OVERALL): REST & REPEAT CYCLE

DAY 31 – 90:

❖ Diet: Refine calorie consumption goals every one to two weeks as needed

❖ Diet: Continue using calorie consumption log book

❖ Exercise: Continue exercise program and advance level(s) if comfortable

BEYOND DAY 90:

❖ Diet: Continue learning and perfecting

❖ Exercise: Continue learning and perfecting

COMPONENT THREE:
STRESS

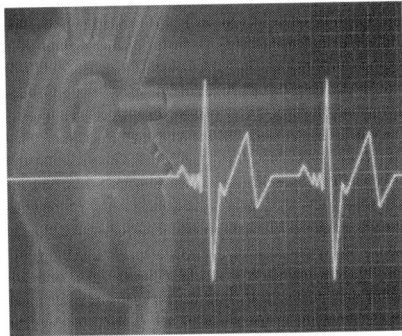

CHAPTER TEN:
EFFECTS OF STRESS—THE YING OR THE YANG?

The concept of stress is not new and it has gained much more attention in recent decades as our lifestyle has grown increasingly hectic. We know now that chronic stress can lead to illness and even endanger our lives. Unfortunately, resources for effective programs dealing with stress modification are often overshadowed by other modifiable health factors such as diet and exercise. For most people, a disparity exists between the recognition of stress and actually applying practical methods of coping with the problem.

Even with a proper diet and exercise routine, our health may be at significant risk if we let daily stress overwhelm us. This component of our program begins with a discussion of the reaction to stress and its various effects. Later, we will discuss many common stressors. In addition to promoting awareness, we will describe methods and techniques of managing and decreasing stress and anxiety.

Stress can affect our health in several ways. First, the actual stress itself can damage our body's immune system and cause disease. We will describe this process in more detail in just a moment.

Next, stress can reduce the effectiveness of our diet and exercise programs, which we know are essential for health. Indirectly, our motivation and resolve to exercise and diet often take a back seat, so to speak, when we are dealing with a difficult situation. In this case, we may feel overwhelmed to the point where proper diet and exercise seem to be more of a burden, rather than a priority.

In a more direct example, stress can alter our normal physiologic processes that affect our other components of health. A few of the many negative associated effects of stress include digestive problems, decreased energy, fatigue and insomnia. All of these symptoms tend to reduce the efficiency of our diet and exercise regimen.

For instance, increased stress levels can interfere with normal digestive patterns causing symptoms of indigestion, constipation and diarrhea. This will often lead to poor absorption of vital dietary nutrients and may even cause mal-nutrition if untreated. Furthermore, stress can lead to fatigue which affects the quality of our exercise and prolongs the recuperation time that is required between workouts.

Again, we see how our four major health components are linked to one another, either to improve or reduce our overall wellness. Combining the stress modification component into our diet and exercise plan can significantly improve our health beyond what is possible when approaching these components in a single fashion.

So what exactly is stress anyhow? We hear this term all the time, but it may not always be clear what constitutes stress or when it actually occurs. To answer that question, we need to define a couple related terms. First, a **stressor** can be defined as a stimulus that increases the demand on an individual. An important work assignment and driving through rush hour traffic are two good examples of common, everyday stressors.

These stressors can lead to an unhealthy stress response, especially in those who do not use proper coping mechanisms. Notice here, that I use the term "unhealthy stress response." This is because at certain times, we may actually benefit from stress. In fact, it is a necessary part of life.

Some of you may have heard of the "fight or flight" response. This is our body's ability to produce adrenaline in times of danger. Adrenaline is one of the major hormones released when dealing with stressful situations. For instance, when you hear a noise at night and fear that someone may be breaking into your home, your adrenaline level immediately rises — this is the "fight or flight" response. A number of important physiologic changes occur when this adrenaline is released, which helps us combat an immediate threat.

Some of these changes include an increase in heart rate, blood pressure and respiratory rate which all facilitate the delivery of oxygen and other nutrients to our bodies. Digestion, on the other hand, is inhibited since it is not needed when dealing with an immediate threat. In other words, adrenaline improves our ability to stand up to a stressful encounter (fight) or run away from it (flight). So you can see that the reaction to stress, in some cases, is a perfectly natural response that may even help to preserve life in certain critical situations.

We have all heard of amazing feats that human beings have demonstrated during times of extreme challenges, such as the man or woman who lifts a particularly heavy object in order to save the life of another person. This is undoubtedly due to the "fight or flight" response. A more common example involves playing sports. Whether you are trying to out run an opponent or hit a homerun, in either case your body produces adrenaline to enhance your performance.

The most important point is that stress is a natural everyday occurrence and how we respond to stress determines whether or not it becomes detrimental to our health. Therefore, the term **stress** can be defined as a given reaction to a situation or stressor. Although we often view stress as an external entity that we have little or no control over, in reality it is actually an internal **response** that can ultimately be controlled by our mind. This point is critical to our understanding of stress management and allows us to better control a given situation or modify our circumstance.

While reading through this book, you may continue to see the common use of the word stress to imply a harmful situation or unwanted stimulus. However, it is important to remember that it is generally our response to stress and our inability to effectively cope with stress that endangers our health, not the actual stressor itself.

So how is it that stress is bad for our health? Well, as you have just learned, stress can release adrenaline, which leads to a number of significant physiologic changes including an increased heart rate and blood pressure. While these responses are perfectly normal and healthy during activities such as exercise, they become detrimental when sustained over long periods.

To explain how this works, let's revisit our favorite car analogy. Our bodies are finely tuned machines similar to modern day automobiles. At times, we need to accelerate our cars in order to avoid a harmful accident or deadly crash, similar to our body's "fight or flight" response.

In addition, our cars are manufactured to withstand normal wear and tear and actually depend on routine use to ensure proper function. Anyone who has stored their auto in a garage for too long and attempts to start it without success can attest to the importance of avoiding prolonged inactivity. Humans also need routine periodic activity that involves a temporary increase in our physiologic demand thru activities that involve both mental concentration and physical activity.

On the other hand, if we continually rev up our engine while driving, we place an unnecessary demand on our vehicle. This can lead to damage and the need for unscheduled maintenance. In a similar way, prolonged stress levels can increase our blood pressure and damage blood vessels which in turn lead to illness such as kidney disease, heart disease and stroke.

To illustrate the significant effect that stress can have on our endocrine hormones, take a look at the following graft. Here we see the "resting" adrenaline level on the very left side of the graft. Immediately to the right of the resting level, a dramatic spike in adrenaline has occurred, typical of a stress induced elevation.

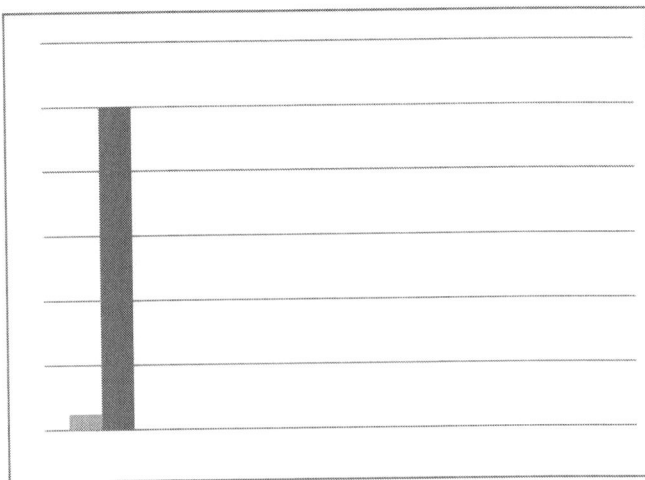

Stress Induced Elevation of Adrenaline

Another central hormone involved in the stress response is cortisol. This hormone is similar to adrenaline in that normal levels are vital for life. Prolonged high levels due to stress, however, can damage our organs and tissues. In addition, abnormal increases in cortisol are thought to play an important role in our susceptibility to infection and may even reduce our defense against cancer.

Most of us have either heard or used an agent that is essentially identical to cortisol. This agent is the drug called cortisone, which often comes in the form of an over-the-counter cream. Cortisone is used to treat many diseases, and its main mechanism of action is to reduce our body's immune cells that cause inflammation such as what occurs in many rashes. Cortisone can also be taken in pill form to treat certain inflammatory lung diseases such as asthma or chronic bronchitis.

One of the undesired effects of absorbing or ingesting too much cortisone is that it can damage our immune system, which is needed to fight infectious diseases and cancers. Therefore, sustained increases in our own production of cortisol, from stress for example, can increase our susceptibility to a variety of illnesses, including cancer.

RESPONDING TO STRESS:

How is it that two individuals facing the same situation can have such different responses? Why is it that a stressor for one individual which causes significant distress can be deemed downright trivial to someone else? There are several reasons to explain this phenomenon.

First, we know that stress is really a reaction or response. This reaction depends partly on our individual personalities. We all meet people who seem like they're always on edge, while others don't appear to have a care in the world. Thus, it is natural that an individual who exhibits an explosive personality will often react in a similar temperamental manner when faced with a challenge.

On the other side, appearances can be deceiving. Some people seem to be very calm and collected on the outside, while internalizing all their negative feelings until they have a nervous breakdown. These individuals may actually feel a great deal of anxiety and worry, without exhibiting overt signs of stress.

In either case, it is important to openly acknowledge our individual personality traits, since they can both hinder or help us cope with stress. For instance, you may feel that you have a tendency to become distracted by seemingly small problems or that everything "stresses you out." If this is the case, it is important to recognize this trait so that you can effectively manage your stress. One important coping method in this specific situation would be to focus on one problem or task at a time without trying to multitask.

On the other hand, you might be someone who has a hard time expressing how you feel. In this case, it would be beneficial to find a person whom you really trust and who can lend an ear. If you tend to internalize all your feelings, you may find a great relief in discussing your stressors with someone else.

No matter what your personality type, the key is to be honest with yourself and acknowledge both your own strengths and weaknesses. Only then will you be able to evaluate how these traits may help or hinder you in managing a stressful situation.

Another reason that people tend to react to the same type of stressor in different ways is due to their prior level of experience. Many times, a lack of knowledge or experience leads to high anxiety. Take, for instance, a person who has undergone several tax audits in his or her lifetime. This individual will likely have a much different perception of this stressor than someone who has never gone through a similar circumstance.

In general, the person who has had previous success dealing with a problem or challenge will often have a calmer reaction to the same challenge in the future. On the other hand, the individual who has had a terrible experience in the past and dreads a similar experience can find relief by shifting their focus away from that memory by concentrating on more positive thoughts.

While it may be true that someone who has had a negative experience in the past, from say a tax audit, may be more apprehensive when facing the same situation, in general, knowledge is power. Taking time to familiarize one's self with a current problem will usually help ameliorate some stress.

Lastly, the magnitude of a given stressor or the number of stressors that we encounter at one time can determine our reaction. Obviously, the person who needs to balance a dozen tasks at once or has had a string of recent misfortunes will likely have a reduced ability to cope with additional stress than someone whose stressors have longer lapses between them.

Learning stress reduction techniques and understanding how to use stress management tools will reduce the negative effects of any stressor on an individual, regardless of his or her personality or the type of stress encountered. Combined with proper diet and exercise, stress reduction can optimize our body's defenses and help prevent or delay the most common human diseases causing illness and death. Combining these healthy components into a daily regimen is by far more powerful than any pill or medical treatment known to man.

CHAPTER ELEVEN:
STRESSORS AND COMMON CAUSES OF STRESS

We can now discuss a number of common stressors that may negatively impact our health. Later, we will address helpful tips and techniques to prevent stress or to modify our responses to common and unexpected stressors.

Common Stressors and Sources of Stress Include:

- ➢ Relationship/Family Stresses:
  - ✓ Divorce
  - ✓ Death of a spouse or loved one
  - ✓ Sexual problems
  - ✓ Infidelity
  - ✓ Envy /jealousy
  - ✓ Newborn birth /newly adopted child
  - ✓ Disabled/sick child
  - ✓ Troubled child/behavior concerns
  - ✓ Financial difficulty/arguments
  - ✓ Chronic illness/injured partner
  - ✓ Moving

➢ Work Related Stresses:
   - ✓ Upcoming deadlines
   - ✓ Loss of a job
   - ✓ Conflict with another employee/colleague
   - ✓ Proposed future layoffs/job cuts/fear of termination
   - ✓ New boss
   - ✓ Relocation
   - ✓ Promotion/added responsibility
   - ✓ Passed over for a raise or expected bonus

➢ Habitual Stresses:
   - ✓ Lack of sleep
   - ✓ Smoking/tobacco use
   - ✓ Excessive alcohol intake/drug abuse
   - ✓ Excessive coffee/caffeinated beverages
   - ✓ Lack of exercise
   - ✓ Poor diet

Obviously this list does not include every stress that we may encounter on a day-to-day basis; however it does list many common and major issues that confront us at one time or another.

In this section we will not discuss family and work related stressors directly. You will find that many of the general techniques and stress management tools provided later in this section, however, are applicable and will assist in coping with these types of stresses as well. The insight that can be gained towards the end of the book in the section on spirituality will also be relevant to many of the family and work related problems that we may encounter in our lives and provide us with tools to address these particular stressors.

Instead, we will focus on what I call habitual stressors — those behaviors or patterns of behavior that are most commonplace and that are most harmful to the majority of readers. These types of stresses can severely harm a person. Unfortunately, even though several of them are among the most important preventable risk factors for disease, they are also some of the hardest patterns to change.

The good news is that we have already addressed two of the more common causes of habitual stress: poor diet and exercise. As we already know, eating a well-balanced diet and getting proper exercise will lead to an improvement in overall health and well-being. Additionally, we also now understand that consuming unhealthy foods, neglecting exercise or excessive overtraining can "stress" our bodies and may lead to significant health problems. Enough said!

SLEEP

Good sleep patterns are another very important habit to establish. It helps us combat fatigue and allows our bodies to undergo vital rejuvenating processes. Like diet and exercise, sleep is often neglected to our own detriment. Lack of appropriate sleep increases the stress on our bodily systems and decreases our ability to cope with outside stressors at the same time. The amount of rest required varies, but in general we should all attempt to dedicate a solid 7-8 hours of sleep per night.

The quality of sleep is just as important as the quantity. In order to maximize the benefits of rest, we need to enter a state of deep sleep call **REM** sleep. Rapid eye movement, or REM, is the period of the sleep cycle when dreaming occurs and which is deeper and more rejuvenating. Don't worry if you can't recall dreaming in the morning since most dreams are forgotten. You should be more concerned, however, if your sleep is frequently interrupted throughout the night, as this may reduce the number of hours that you spend in REM sleep and therefore cut into your body's opportunity for true rest and rejuvenation.

Insomnia can be manifested in several ways. The problem may be falling asleep, staying asleep throughout the night or waking up too early in the morning. Chronic snoring or gasping during sleep can also seriously affect the quality of sleep and often leads to daytime sleepiness and fatigue. While these problems may be related to an underlying medical issue, much more commonly it is due to poor habits such as excessive alcohol intake or overeating and obesity.

One of the most common errors that we make is to consume caffeinated beverages within several hours of going to bed. A single soft drink, coffee or cup of tea has enough caffeine to make it difficult to initiate sleep. Although green tea has important antioxidants and is often thought to be a healthy alternative to black tea, it still contains some caffeine and may affect your sleep if consumed in large amounts or too late in the day.

Eating right before going to bed can also negatively affect sleep. You should give your body at least a few hours to digest its food prior to lying down; otherwise you risk reflux (heartburn) and indigestion. This was also mentioned in the last section on exercise. Resting after a meal can contribute to weight gain, since our metabolism and ability to burn calories slows considerably during sleep.

The consumption of alcohol prior to bed time can lead to a reduced quality of sleep as well. In addition, some people mistakenly use alcohol or sleeping pills over an extended period of time to help them sleep. Both of these chemicals can make it easier to fall asleep since they cause drowsiness by depressing your central nervous system. However, they often make it difficult to achieve a deep state of sleep and can actually lead to chronic fatigue. Thus the use of these substances may be counterproductive in the long run, not to mention they are often habit forming.

A good sleep pattern to establish is to go to bed at approximately the same time each day. Set your alarm or try waking up at the same time each day, too. These are important habits that retrain your biorhythms and set up a consistent cycle, thus improving the quality and quantity of sleep.

Anxiety or stress itself often leads to insomnia, which creates a perpetual cycle of fatigue and stress. In order to combat the problem, we must break this cycle with stress reduction techniques that we will soon cover. Some methods that help shift your focus away from anxious thoughts include reading a book or newspaper, or practicing meditation.

Exercise also helps us relax, however it should not be done within an hour or two of sleep. Endorphins and other hormones such as adrenaline released during exercise may actually make falling asleep more difficult if performed before bedtime. Therefore, exercise several hours prior to sleep or earlier in the day if possible.

ALCOHOL

We have already discussed how excessive alcohol can cause insomnia and fatigue, thus making it more difficult to cope with stress. On the one hand, there is a reasonable amount of scientific data to suggest that a *moderate* amount of certain kinds of alcohol may have some health benefits. Most of the studies that show a possible benefit refer to the consumption of red wine (sorry beer and whiskey drinkers.) Furthermore, red wine contains certain chemicals that may reduce our production of bad cholesterol which can lead to heart disease.

However, it is unclear how much one needs to consume in order to have a significant health benefit. It is also unclear which type of red wine is most beneficial, as some types do not seem to protect our heart. Of course drinking any alcohol to excess could damage the heart. Therefore, the possible benefit of moderate red wine consumption must be tempered by the known harmful effects.

To summarize, certain types of red wine **may** help lower the risk of heart disease when consumed in a moderate and responsible manner. However, there are many other types of activities and healthy alternatives that greatly protect the heart without the known risks of alcohol. Therefore, I would caution anyone against using alcohol for reasons related to health.

Most importantly, if you do drink occasionally, moderation is an absolute necessity to prevent undue stress and significant harm to your body. A moderate amount would be no more than one or perhaps two (at the most) measures in a 24 hour period. The definition of a measure is a standard shot of liquor, a 12 ounce beer or a single glass of wine. Thus one beer, one shot or one glass of wine would fall into the category of moderate consumption.

Heavy consumption, on the other hand can cause several types of cancer as well as damage to multiple organs and bodily tissues including your brain, heart, liver, pancreas, digestive tract and nerves to name just a few. Now that's stressful just thinking about it!

SMOKING

Another legal substance that causes a similar amount of stress and damage to our body (or possibly more) is tobacco. This includes both smoking and smokeless products such as chewing tobacco. Nicotine is a drug in tobacco products that can cause effects that are similar to caffeine, but with a much greater potential for addiction.

Both nicotine and caffeine have a similar effect to adrenaline. Recall, adrenaline is the hormone which causes our "fight or flight" response. Basically, all these chemicals keep us on edge — so to speak — by causing an increase in our heart rate and blood pressure, among other things. This forces our heart to work harder and leads to unnecessary physiologic stress. Unlike adrenaline, however, caffeine and nicotine cause an artificially *prolonged* stress response since it takes many hours to rid them from our bodies. This effect is unhealthy and over time may damage our bodies.

Worst by far is that tobacco products and cigarette smoke contains literally hundreds of damaging toxins. These chemicals are extremely harmful to multiple organs and tissues, not to mention their excellent ability to cause cancer. The risk of oral and lung cancer is significantly elevated with smoking and chronic tobacco use. In fact, one of the leading causes of death in the United States is lung cancer, which in most cases is associated with smoking. If that's not a true stressor then I don't know what is!

Combining alcohol and smoking together can potentiate each product's negative effects leading to a much higher risk of health problems. For example, both alcohol and smoking are known to increase the risk of oral and throat cancer independent of one another. For someone who both smokes and drinks, his or her potential risk, then, is not just twice as high as someone who indulges in one of these. His or her risk factor is actually exponentially higher. So, alcohol and tobacco work together to destroy our health in the same exponential manner that our Healthy 4 components work together to strengthen our overall health. Thus, these habitual stressors should be avoided for their obvious health risks.

So far we have discussed how stress reduction can involve both the abstinence of specific harmful habits as well as a modification of other habits to promote healthy living. In the next chapter, we will review a variety of simple yet effective tools and methods of coping with stress on a daily basis.

CHAPTER TWELVE:
STRESS REDUCTION—TIPS AND TECHNIQUES

CONTROLLED BREATHING:

When feeling increased anxiety or stress it is often helpful to perform breathing exercises. With this technique, take a slow and steady deep breath through your nose and exhale in a similar controlled fashion through your mouth. Do not hold your breath at any point. Rather, spend a few minutes focusing your attention on controlling the rate and depth of your breathing. It should feel natural and relaxing, slow and deliberate – deep and not shallow. Keep your thoughts centered on the movement of air in and out of your body. This will create calm and shifts focus away from stressful images or thoughts.

It is best to do this in a quiet area if possible. You may wish to close your eyes as this can sometimes help to avoid certain visual distractions. Either way, this simple tool can be used at any time, even if you only have a minute or two to spare.

VISUALIZATION:

This technique is often incorporated with controlled breathing or can be performed on its own. In this context, visualization means that you focus all your attention onto a chosen mental image that may relax you or assist you in overcoming a challenging situation.

For instance, some people may choose a warm tropical island with beautiful turquoise water and soft, pure white sand as their mental destination. The more specific or detailed your image, the more real it becomes, lending itself to greater relaxation. In the tropical island example, try to imagine specifics such as a gentle breeze against your face or the soft, silky grains caressing your feet as you move them back and forth in the sand. Again, you will want to avoid noisy areas. It works best if you can find a quiet place where you can close your eyes or free yourself from obvious distraction.

Other images may be the picture of your child's smiling face perhaps or a quiet mountain stream. The number of images you can come up with are endless. It could be a setting that is familiar to you already or one that is completely made up. The key is to choose a mental picture that is both pleasing and relaxing for you.

Another form of visualization, in contrast, requires you to think of the particular challenge or stressful situation. This is most useful when dealing with performance based tasks that are causing an increased level of anxiety. For instance, a surgeon preparing for a complex case will visualize the operation, going through each step one by one in his or her head to build confidence.

Another example would be public speaking or a work presentation. In this scenario, it is helpful to visualize yourself on stage or it front of an audience presenting your material in a relaxed and composed manner. Try to think of possible challenges that you may face, and then use positive visualization to come up with the solutions. In this way, your visual preparation will reduce the anxiety associated with a difficult task.

MEDITATION:

In a manner of speaking, we have broached the subject of meditation already through visualization and controlled breathing techniques. These are commonly used in the practice of meditation. There are many forms of meditation and different philosophies that are ascribed to each of these forms. To keep it simple however, meditation implies that you remove all negative thoughts and focus or concentrate your mind in a more productive way. Often this concentration can be on a single object or sound.

It requires discipline to focus the mind and free your thoughts from distractions. In fact, Buddhist Monks often spend many years developing and mastering this technique. It is a widely held belief in Eastern Cultures that peace, harmony and transformation of the mind are achieved through this practice.

When practicing meditation, again it's important to find a quiet place free of interruptions. You will want to allocate a larger amount of free time for this activity. If your time is limited, use the simpler techniques of controlled breathing and visual imagery instead, as they are more practical for short term needs.

Begin by sitting in a comfortable position, however avoid a lazy posture or relaxed position that could make you tired or lose focus. Try to clear your mind completely of any negative images or scattered thoughts. You may find that this is actually quite difficult, especially at first.

Several images and thoughts tend to pop in and out of our consciousness despite our best efforts. This is not surprising, as most of us are accustomed to a fast pace world that conditions our mind to constantly race back and forth to keep up with the demands of everyday life. It will take effort, but with practice you can train your mind to let go of many of these thoughts during meditation. When unwanted images do occur, the simple act of refocusing your concentration away from all your stress is soothing and relaxing.

If you're having trouble clearing your mind, it helps to develop and practice a **mantra**. A mantra for all practical purposes is an expression, syllable, phrase or vocalization that helps to focus one's mind and creates calm during meditation. It is a tool for freeing your mind from negative thoughts and allows you to focus on an object that creates peace and harmony. The actual sound does not necessarily need to have meaning to others but it helps to have meaning or purpose to those who use it.

A common mantra used by Buddhists in Tibet is "Om Mani Padme Hum" which conveys great meaning to those who use it. Another mantra that has religious meaning could be "God is great," for example. Again, it is not necessary for it to be religious. It doesn't even need to be an actual word or phrase. It is simply a vocal expression that brings you closer to peace and harmony.

Whatever mantra you choose, be sure to repeat it slowly, focusing on the sound or phrase. Furthermore, do not be self conscious when performing this verbalization when you first start practicing. Remember, your quest is to improve your health and well-being which is always a noble pursuit and thus should be free of self criticism or self consciousness. Millions of people around the world routinely practice this art without thought of self. I encourage you to give it a try at some point. You just may surprise yourself.

Utilizing the breathing techniques and visualization methods previously described are practical, too, and are a great place to begin basic stress reduction. However, for a more advanced and deeper level of calm, there are few things that compare to regular meditation and mastering this art will help us achieve our long-term goals of overall stress reduction.

Although most of us are not in training to become monks and our goal is not necessarily to seek enlightenment, I do recommend learning more about this valuable age-old technique. There are numerous books and articles on this subject. The writings of the Dalai Lama of Tibet on meditation and transforming the mind are excellent reads and are translated in a way that is both philosophical and practical.

HARNESSING YOUR SOCIAL NETWORK:

Simply talking with someone you love or trust about your stress can also be a very cathartic and calming experience. As we have previously discussed, allowing your stressors to build up without finding an outlet to relieve some of your anxiety will likely result in harm over the long run. One way to relieve stress is to ask for advice or simply accept another person's willingness to lend an ear. You should never feel guilt during this process. Asking for help is *never* a sign of weakness; rather it shows your courage and resolve to better yourself or improve your situation.

Above all, be honest with yourself and try to minimize defensive reactions, especially if you feel you are being criticized. Remember that we all have our strengths and weaknesses. Constructive dialogue may involve suggestions regarding self improvement that you may not have considered previously. However, it should never involve passing judgment or feelings of guilt. Therefore, it is import to talk to someone you trust or respect.

Some resources in your immediate network may include:

➢ A best friend
➢ Spouse
➢ Parent or sibling

> ➤ Religious leader or teacher at your place of worship
> ➤ Your doctor
> ➤ A Colleague or counselor at work

Other possible resources to consider include:
> ➤ Specific interest or self help groups
> ➤ Social worker
> ➤ Therapist or psychologist specializing in stress management

It is important to remind yourself that you are not alone. You have people in the world, whether familiar or unfamiliar, who love you or simply want to help you. You may find solace in the fact that others have similar stresses. Additionally you can discover a new method of addressing a particular problem. Either way, you have little to lose and often much to gain by expressing your concerns with others who want to help.

FINDING A NEW HOBBY OR SPEICAL INTEREST:

Sometimes stress occurs when we spend too much time on one particular activity or become too single minded in our pursuits. Beginning a new hobby may be just the answer in this case. Developing new interests and skills builds self confidence and may improve your ability to cope with other challenging tasks or stressors. Additionally, it focuses your attention on something enjoyable and productive.

It may seem like common sense, but think twice before participating in an activity that causes you additional stress. For instance, if you have a fear of heights, it may not be an opportune time to take flight lessons when you feel you are dealing with significant stress. On the one hand, conquering your fears can be a very liberating experience. However, you need to assess your current stress level and decide if it's in your best interest to take on a new challenge. The key is to find a new hobby that is both motivating and relaxing at the same time. The choice is up to you. Here are just a few suggestions:

✓ Building models (such as cars, trains, planes)
✓ Making clothes or knitting
✓ Gardening

✓ Fishing or hunting
✓ Taking a cooking class
✓ Joining a league (such as soft ball or bowling)
✓ Enrolling in a book club
✓ Volunteering (such as in a shelter or after school/big brother programs)
✓ Trying a new sport (such as golf or tennis)
✓ Bird watching
✓ Painting
✓ Taking a pottery class
✓ Writing
✓ Doing crossword or jigsaw puzzles
✓ Reading for pleasure

The possibilities are nearly limitless. Spend some time thinking about something you would like to try first. If it seems interesting and plausible then go for it. Finding a true passion often involves trial and error, so don't be afraid to give something a try and don't fret if it doesn't work out — just move on to something new and interesting. Life is about learning and developing your interests and talents. This process doesn't end after your formal education is completed but continues throughout your entire life.

POSTURAL TECHNIQUES:

This category includes the common practices of Tai Chi and Yoga. Tai Chi is actually a form of Chinese martial arts which focuses on certain body posture and movements that create harmony with the mind and body and bring about calm. Yoga similarly focuses on posture and body movements and may have a similar calming effect.

Millions of people around the world practice these types of exercises and have found them helpful. Teaching all of these techniques is obviously well beyond the scope of this book. Taking a class is highly recommended. As with so many other things, a wealth of knowledge can be found on the internet regarding these specific stress reductions techniques.

In the meantime, a simple exercise you can try on your own is to stand in an upright position focusing on keeping your spine straight. Next push your arms out from the center of your body slowly in a controlled fashion. The focus should be on breathing throughout these movements. Never hold your breath. Once your arms are fully extended in front of you, pause for a moment before retracting your arms in a similar controlled manner.

Breathing should never be labored. You can try "abdominal breathing" which is a deeper, slow controlled breathing technique that seems to come from your diaphragm. By concentrating on the movement of your diaphragm and abdomen (which is below your rib cage) rather than your chest, your breath will seem deeper and this may increase your state of relaxation.

Many routine stretching exercises can have a similar effect of promoting relaxation. They usually do not require the acquisition of new knowledge and can be used immediately to help reduce your stress level. Most importantly, like all postural exercises, stretching exercise should be performed in a controlled fashion without sudden or jerky movements. Proper breathing is still required and will help facilitate oxygen and blood flow to your muscles and connective tissues. Refer to our website: www.Healthy4.com for more information on proper stretching and postural movements.

BIOFEEDBACK:

This technique basically involves monitoring certain quantifiable bodily functions to improve awareness of stress and its effects on the body. For example, instruments or monitors can be used to examine your heart rate and blood pressure during times of stress and relaxation. By linking these vital functions during periods of stress and calm we may be able to promote a greater awareness and control of stress.

A simple way to begin experimenting with biofeedback would be manually monitoring your pulse rate. The pulse rate is another term for heart rate: it refers to how fast your heart beats and is measured by the number of beats per minute. A **normal** resting adult heart rate should fall between **60 and 100 beats per minute.**

Blood pressure, on the other hand, is the actual pressure that our blood exerts on the walls of our arteries as blood flows through the circulatory system. A **normal blood pressure** is < **120/80** while a high blood pressure is defined as blood pressure > 140/90. Some of you may be wondering why we having two numbers for blood pressure. The first number is the pressure that our blood exerts in our artery at the moment the heart is contracting. The second number is the pressure that our blood exerts in our artery at the moment when the heart relaxes.

You can use biofeedback to measure your own vital signs at various times during the day to provide important feedback or information to help you assess and reduce your stress at a given time.

To check your heart rate manually, check your pulse at the wrist by using a watch with a second hand. Count the number of beats that you feel over 15 seconds and multiply this number by 4 to obtain the number of beats per minute. To check blood pressure, however, you will need to purchase an automated blood pressure monitor at your local pharmacy or retail health store.

Our blood pressure and heart rate typically increase during times of stress. Thus, monitoring these variations provide us with another source of information regarding our state of anxiety. Keep in mind that there are other factors besides stress that will elevate blood pressure and heart rate.

Take for instance our discussion on the habitual stressors: caffeine and nicotine. If you are a smoker or drink coffee prior to using biofeedback techniques, you will likely see an elevation in your vital signs. In this case, it would be unclear how much of this elevation is due to the absorbed chemicals and how much can be attributable to a specific anxiety. Nevertheless, it would help you to assess how this stress is affecting your bodily functions.

Some people find biofeedback particularly useful, while others may not feel a significant benefit. In either case, since knowledge is power, I have included this method as one more tool for you to try if you wish.

COGNITIVE THERAPY:

This term refers to treatment that targets the way you think. It is sometimes offered by mental health specialists as a means to change a specific behavior. However, you can use these thought changing techniques yourself to help view a particular stressor in a healthier way or reduce the effect of the stressor.

This process involves creating a positive internal monologue. In other words, by telling yourself to look at the bright side, things actually do become brighter. This does not mean that you should lie to yourself. Rather, it is a way to keep problems in perspective and to usher in more positive thinking.

We know that happy people generally feel less stressed and more in control than those who are depressed. Does this mean that people who are happy have less challenges or stressors than those than those who have a cynical view of the world? Of course not! It's often a simple case of mind over matter. Never underestimate the power of positive thought!

When stress occurs, we have the choice to view it on a continuum that goes from the worst to the best case scenario. If we always think to our self that the world is going to end, sadly it may be a self-fulfilling prophecy. However, if we begin to search for the positive side of every experience, we soon find that we have more control over our own destiny. We all have the ability to modify our thoughts. Like so many other important aspects of life, this takes frequent effort and practice, but it ultimately pays off.

I will admit that some events and situations are in fact very stressful and cause enormous pain. Positive thinking may not always diminish the weight of your problems and at certain moments in life it may be extremely difficult to see the bright side of anything. However, the more often we avoid negativity and replace it with positive thinking, the better we are able to cope with stress regardless of the magnitude.

Here are some examples of positive phrases and their negative counterparts:

POSITIVE PHRASES:	NEGATIVE PHRASES:
1) I CAN do this	I can't do it
2) Things WILL get better	It won't get better
3) It's NOT that bad	It's really bad
4) I AM going to feel better	What if it doesn't get better
5) I AM capable	I am unable
6) I WILL get through this	I can't handle this
7) This is a challenge	I hate this
8) Tomorrow WILL be better	I'll never feel better
9) Things could be worse	This is the worst
10) I am still blessed	I am so unlucky

You can see that the way we choose to think about something can significantly affect our motivation and our ability to handle a given problem. Write down some positive phrases for yourself and try repeating them over and over again in times of stress. You will soon find that your ability to cope with stress improves, and your entire outlook will likely become more positive as well.

STRESS AVOIDANCE:

Stress is a common part of life and many times we cannot escape from it. Procrastination prolongs the inevitable and may compound the problem. In some cases avoiding a stressful situation is just plain irresponsible and dangerous. Take for instance a recent worrisome change in health or unexplained medical problem. In this scenario, one should never try to forget about the problem and avoid seeing the doctor. Some situations demand that you face your stress head on.

Other situations are not as critical and simply avoiding a stressor may be the healthier choice. For example, spending time in rush hour traffic can be very frustrating and stressful for some people. If this is the case, or in times when you are particularly stressed, it may be more productive to stay at work for another hour and avoid the stressor. Another option would be to spend some time exercising while waiting for traffic to lessen.

EXERCISE:

Lastly, exercise is an excellent way to reduce stress and promote a sense of well-being. As you know now, exercise is one of the four key components of our Healthy 4 plan. We have already discussed a number of the dependent relationships that exist between diet and exercise. It is the same with exercise and stress. Exercising reduces stress and anxiety. In a reciprocal manner, stress reduction improves our ability to exercise by reducing fatigue and increasing our energy levels.

Similarly, diet can affect our exercise and stress level. Consuming too much caffeine in our diet can heighten our physical stress. Furthermore, a dietary protein deficiency would negatively affect our exercise capacity and ability to recuperate. You see where I am going with this! To ensure maximum health and the best bang for your buck, so to speak, you must follow a routine which incorporates all of these components into your present lifestyle.

Your approach to stress management should be similar to dieting and exercise. This is to say, coping with stress requires a lifelong dedication and frequent application of stress management techniques.

It's time to review all of the stress management techniques discussed in this section and incorporate them into our overall program. Unlike the exercise component of this program, you can incorporate these tools right away into your routine, beginning with the first 15 days of our Healthy 4 plan.

HEALTHY 4 SUMMARY PLAN FOR DIET, EXERCISE AND STRESS:

<u>DAY 1 – DAY 15:</u>

- ❖ Diet: Begin recording your daily calorie consumption each day for the first 15 days (review the nutrition labels)

- ❖ Exercise Program: None (continue with your normal activity and routine)

- ❖ Stress Management Tips and Techniques:
  - ✓ Find time to utilize visualization
  - ✓ Control your breathing
  - ✓ Try meditation
  - ✓ Use postural techniques: such as tai chi, yoga or routine stretching
  - ✓ Access your social network and talk with others
  - ✓ Start a new hobby
  - ✓ Use biofeedback
  - ✓ Ensure adequate sleep
  - ✓ Reduce caffeine and alcohol intake
  - ✓ Avoid tobacco
  - ✓ Exercise
  - ✓ Maintain a proper diet
  - ✓ Avoid the stressor if appropriate
  - ✓ Focus on positive thoughts/develop a healthy internal monologue

<u>DAY 16 – DAY 30:</u>

- ❖ Diet: Continue recording your daily calorie consumption and use this information to establish a daily calorie consumption limit (such as 2000 calories)

- ❖ Diet: Use the following dieting pearls to assist you:
  - ✓ Avoid eating until full
  - ✓ Eat small portions or reduce your meal size
  - ✓ Eat *more* frequently during the day versus one or two large meals
  - ✓ Don't wait until your hunger is strong before you eat
  - ✓ **Slow down** when you eat
  - ✓ Pack your own food and carry nutritional supplements with you
  - ✓ Avoid eating as a reflex to hunger (assess for abnormal cues)
  - ✓ Avoid buffets and all-you-can-eat menus
  - ✓ Consume low calorie foods and drinks
  - ✓ Count your calories and set daily goals
  - ✓ Keep yourself well hydrated
  - ✓ Drink water rather high calorie drinks
  - ✓ Try a healthy snack *before* a meal
  - ✓ Forget about adhering to traditional course meals (i.e. 3 or 4 courses)
  - ✓ DON'T feel the need to clear your plate and STOP eating once you meet your dietary goals
  - ✓ Never eat before going to sleep
  - ✓ Associate positive thought to healthy foods
  - ✓ Eat a well-balanced diet
  - ✓ Consume most of your fats from unsaturated, non-trans fat sources
  - ✓ Don't prepare or cover your food with unhealthy toppings

- ❖ Exercise Program: Start beginner level one program

<u>Day 1 (DAY 16 OVERALL):</u>

Cardio training: **30 minutes** elliptical machine, swimming, stationary bike or equivalent

Core resistance training: push ups and/or bench press **2 sets**

Core resistance training: pull ups and/or pull downs **2 sets**

Sit ups: **2 sets**

Day 2 (DAY 17 OVERALL): Rest

Day 3 (DAY 18 OVERALL):
 Cardio training: **30 minutes** elliptical machine, swimming,
  stationary bike or equivalent
 Core resistance training: squats **2 sets**
 Sit ups: **2 sets**

Day 4 (DAY 19 OVERALL): Rest

Day 5 (DAY 20 OVERALL):

 Cardio training: **30 minutes**
 Core resistance training: push ups and/or bench press **2 sets**
 Core resistance training: pull ups and/or pull downs **2 sets**
 Sit ups **2 sets**

Day 6 & 7 (DAY 21 & 22 OVERALL): REST & REPEAT CYCLE

❖ Stress Management: Continue using tips and techniques

Day 31 – 90:

❖ Diet: Refine calorie consumption goals every one to two weeks
 as needed

❖ Exercise: Continue exercise program and advance level(s) if
 comfortable

❖ Stress Management: Continue using tips and techniques

<u>Beyond Day 90:</u>

❖ Diet: Continue lifelong learning and perfecting

❖ Exercise: Continue lifelong learning and perfecting

❖ Stress Management: Continue lifelong learning and perfection

COMPONENT FOUR:
SPIRITUALITY

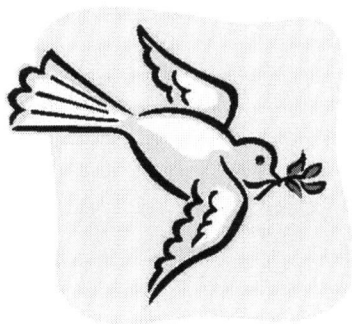

CHAPTER THIRTEEN:
THE MEANING OF
SPIRITUALITY

Well, we have made it to the fourth and final principle component of the Healthy 4 program, spirituality. We have discussed many issues and provided significant knowledge concerning dietary, exercise and stress reduction practices. The first three sections dealt with facets of health that are more intuitive and most commonly addressed in the media. This last section, however, may be more difficult to grasp at first glance. Nevertheless, it's equally as vital to our wellness. Most importantly, integrating spiritual thoughts and practices into your daily routine will optimize health and create peace in your life.

Unfortunately, many people view this topic in terms of black and white. Some individuals view spirituality too rigidly, as a way of soliciting religion perhaps. Others may feel that it's an abstract concept and fail to see its practicality. To find the meaning of spirituality, we must first set aside our own attitudes or biases in order to prevent them from interfering with our quest to gain insight and knowledge.

Let's begin by examining what spirituality implies. This word may have several different meanings depending on the context in which it is used. Religion is often used synonymously with spirituality. Followers of a specific religion often do feel spiritually fulfilled through the practice of their faith. It can be argued, however, that one does not necessarily have to be religious to be considered a spiritual person. In this case, the word may be used in a more esoteric sense. Here, we may presume that such a person has transcended from the material world and has found deeper meaning and existence. In a sense, they have become enlightened.

Perhaps the most practical application of spirituality is used to describe those who have found their calling or sense of purpose. And for the purposes of the Healthy 4 program, we will consider spirituality neither as religion or enlightenment but rather a sense of well-being and purpose. In this case, we become more than our superficial possessions and material thoughts. To find purpose in one's life is the essence of living. Without it we feel lost and uncertain. We must all discover our sense of purpose to find peace and joy; otherwise we can never be truly healthy, let alone happy.

We all have variable interests and pursuits, and each finds his or her purpose in different ways. Thus, no person can tell you or me what our individual purpose is or should be in life. There is no road map or exact guide for this quest. We must all find our own direction and calling. Some people are fortunate to find their calling early in life. Others never appear to know what they are searching for at all. What is most important is that we seek the answers with open eyes and an open mind.

The purpose is to become healthier, and ultimately we need to do it for not only ourselves but for others. Being spiritual, then, is about honoring an entity greater than ourselves – not only God, but others, too.

Essentially we need to be healthy not only for ourselves (to feel good) but also for those who are close to us, such as family, so we will live longer and be able to care for them as their needs require. Beyond the scope of our own circle of friends and family, we need to be healthy for the whole of society: to not be a drain on resources and to set a positive example to others so they may benefit from our good health.

True purpose in the mind brings about purposeful actions. Of course, many things bring pleasure and gratification. However, when honestly viewing one's life at critical stages of development, one must feel a sense of purpose or meaning in order to attain true calm and internal peace as well as to avoid anxiety, despair or depression.

The methods of obtaining this peace (and thus mental health) vary but all have a common theme: they involve deeds aimed at helping or benefiting others. Some use prayer to attain peace and well-being. Others obtain their sense of purpose by helping their children become good people. Yet others volunteer a large part of their time and energy, despite having little financial reward and minimum materialistic gain.

The following chapter will discuss in greater details some means of achieving spirituality and, particularly, our sense of purpose.

Once we feel we have found purpose, however, our quest does not end. Similar to our dedication towards diet, exercise and stress management, spirituality is a lifelong pursuit. We must continually incorporate and modify practices that support our own sense of purpose to ensure our future well-being.

Although spirituality is the fourth vital component that is essential for health and life, most of us tend to minimize or neglect this area when approaching our physical health. Relegated to the self-help section, spirituality has arbitrarily been separated from discussions on weight loss, exercise or diet in many typical wellness programs. However, these important individual aspects of physical health will ultimately weaken without incorporating spirituality.

Achieving our true physical and mental health potential is only possible when we include spirituality into the other major components that we have covered so far. There is much scientific evidence to support this, too, and for those wishing to read more on the relationship between health and spirituality, I encourage you to visit our website at Healthy4.com.

CHAPTER FOURTEEN: DEVELOPING YOUR SPIRITUAL SIDE

To find our spirituality, it becomes important to take a step back and reflect on what it is not. As previously stated, spirituality in essence can be defined as one's sense of purpose. We also know that we may follow different avenues in our pursuit of spiritual awakening. Of course, sometimes we are blissfully unaware that we are on the wrong road. That is, until we realize at some point that something is wrong or we feel lost.

THE QUEST FOR MONEY:

Many people look to a chosen career as a place for fulfillment. But often, we are more lost than fulfilled. When we believe that we are not following our true passions, we become frustrated and burned out. In other cases, we may be quite driven to succeed but for the wrong reasons. In both of these circumstances, financial reward often is or becomes the main objective.

Although some may say that the "purpose" of their work is to be financially secure, I argue that this is only a pursuit. What's the difference? A purpose has meaning or value itself, while a pursuit is a means to end. In this case, working for financial security has no meaning by itself. Rather, it is a pursuit towards another goal or some other purpose. The quest for money or financial security alone never leads to a sense of purpose.

The acquisition of money can be a legitimate motivating factor in our lives. From a practical point of view, it is necessary to pay the bills and function in modern society. Unfortunately, we often come to believe that the security of money will bring needed peace and happiness. When financial gain becomes the central focus of our life, the end result is desperation and depression rather than a sense of well-being.

In this frame of mind any attainment of wealth perpetuates the desire for more. It is a temporary gratification and, once a certain standard of living is achieved, a new financial objective is sought and the cycle repeats. This is because wealth does not provide a sense of purpose and the cycle will continue until we truly understand that money by itself does not bring happiness.

That is not to say the acquisition of financial wealth should not be a concern or a pursuit. It is a social reality and obligation to pay for certain necessities in life. Without it, one could not afford a place to live, clothes, transportation and all the other costs of living. Additionally, enjoying financial security and being able to treat yourself to nice things on occasion can be quite pleasurable. But that makes money the means to an end – the pursuit – and not an end itself, which is purpose.

In many ways our culture has trained us to become beholden to money. Like a slave we can become trapped or confined by allowing money to be our master. To free our self from this tyranny, we need to constantly search for deeper meaning in our pursuits. We can do this by asking ourselves on a regular basis, why is it that we want to earn a certain amount of money. If the first answer that pops into your head is that you want to be happier or more at peace, then it is time to re-examine our life's purpose.

BALANCING WORK AND FAMILY:

What about our desire to take care of family and loved ones? That certainly is a worthy objective which can lead to a sense of purpose. However, we must always be honest with ourselves when evaluating our true desire for financial security and re-examine our priorities to ensure that our pursuits do not interfere with our true objective and sense of purpose.

Let's look at the example of providing for family in more detail. A person may feel unfulfilled by their work but continue to do it in order to provide the basic necessities of life that are essential for the well-being of their family. In this case, even those who dislike their job can feel a sense of purpose through their work, since it benefits their families. Or we may want to provide a more comfortable life, such as a nice vacation or a larger house. These aspirations can be worthy pursuits in the right circumstance. However, they can also be a diversion from our main objective.

For instance, what if a person who works hard to provide a "better life" for his or her family comes home constantly disgruntled or distant from their family? In this case, the pursuit may actually be interfering with the true objective. In other words, the pursuit of increased financial security for the purpose of their family's well-being, may in fact be causing more harm than good. Either the individual or the work itself needs to change to ensure the well-being of the family and to reestablish the individual's true sense of purpose.

What's most important is to ask ourselves if our quest for financial gain or our career goals are actually benefiting others or are they truly an attempt to benefit ourselves. I re-emphasize that pursuing money or personal fulfillment is not necessarily bad or unhealthy. The problem occurs when financial gain or career advancement becomes our principle focus, such as the quest for personal power or prestige. When this happens, we lose sight of helping others.

However, when career and financial advancement fosters our ability to help others and facilitates our desire to acquire new skills, that kind of personal gain positively affects those around us. We are filled with a greater sense of purpose and others benefit by our personal growth.

If you dislike your job or career, do not assume making more money will bring you or your family more happiness or contentment. Try to find any aspects of your work that bring joy to others. Make personal connections. This could be as simple as smiling or greeting another person. Helping out a co-worker or doing a good job to help your organization or others ultimately will help create long term mental and spiritual health.

On the other hand, never helping others at work because you are dissatisfied, self absorbed, or wish to be viewed as the best by your employers will eventually cause problems. In the short run, such behavior may lead to career advancement, more power and greater financial gain; however, because the behavior is linked to selfish thinking, it will ultimately lead to despair.

Working against our purpose and behaving in ways that serve only our self will almost certainly lead to such things as divorce, midlife crises, alcoholism or just hidden depression. Never underestimate the good that simple acts of kindness can do – both for others and for your personal well-being.

Ultimately, no matter what job you choose or what your financial objective, you must always try to think and act in ways that benefit others. Granted, it's not always easy, especially when constantly juggling many things at once. However, helping others will lead to an enduring sense of purpose, instead of a temporary and fleeting gratification.

BUILDING RELATIONSHIPS:

As mentioned, strengthening your bond with family members or friends involves considering the well-being of others even before considering your own well-being. Although we sometimes tend to think of our relationships with close family members or friends as stable, requiring perhaps less effort than others, in reality these relationships require continual effort and consideration.

We may think we know how others feel, especially those we live with or work with on a day-to-day basis. We tend to create biases and stereotypes about others that simplify how we view our relationships. The reality, however, is that humans are complex beings and we are all evolving throughout life whether we realize it or not.

Thus, we need to keep an open mind when communicating or interacting with all people. One of the most damaging behaviors to a relationship occurs when we close our mind and assume that we know how others feel without actually asking them in a caring and considerate manner.

It is important to understand that we all have strengths and weaknesses. We often lump people into general groups such as good, bad, kind or mean. In truth, we all have good and bad qualities alike and our behavior is expressed on a large continuum, changing frequently according to our level of stress or life situation.

It is very easy for us to find faults that may or may not exist in our friends, family members or co-workers. It is more difficult however for us to remain open minded and to accept others without being critical, and to focus on the positive qualities each person brings into our life.

Occasionally, we do meet people in our life that we do not see eye to eye with, and we may try to distance ourselves from them. Nevertheless, it is equally important that we give them the benefit of doubt whenever possible and to try to see the world from their point of view, even if we happen to disagree. There is a wrong way and a right way to disagree. The worst way to show disagreement is through intimidation, humiliation or disrespect.

Every once in a while we meet people who just "rub us the wrong way." There may be no accounting for this. Still, it is vital to treat them with respect and communicate openly. This fosters the best possible situation and prevents further deterioration and stress between the parties involved. Most importantly, it creates an internal calm and peace within you that leads to a healthier outlook on mankind, which is a prerequisite to spirituality and optimal wellness.

In addition to mutual respect and open-mindedness, we must also dedicate quality time to others to build our relationships. I mention "quality time" because we not only need to spend an adequate amount of time but we also need to find time to engage in activities and interactions that are beneficial to others as well as ourselves.

For example, a family that sits at the dinner table together engaging one another in meaningful conversation, taking a genuine interest in one another, is spending quality time. On the other hand, if we ignore others by distracting ourselves with busywork or multi-media, we tend to neglect our relationships.

In today's busy world – with its seemingly infinite number of distractions – it is very easy to let our personal relationships fall by the wayside. There is nothing more important than these relationships and we need to make every attempt to regain control of our life by maintaining healthier bonds with our family, friends and loved ones. Thus, we can all find time to put down our cell phones, computers or work during certain periods for the benefit of our relationships. In doing so, we will find greater spirituality and ultimately improved wellness.

RELIGION, PRAYER AND MEDITATION:

From our previous discussion, we can see that spirituality involves thinking or acting in a way that benefits others, rather than our own self. This does not mean that we must neglect all of our own basic needs. Instead, it involves doing something for another entity or being, rather than for the purpose of our own gratification. In doing so, we discover that there is higher significance and meaning beyond our self and thus our spirituality grows.

In these terms, it becomes clear that one can never elevate money higher than one's self or someone else. Although we may try, it's not possible to find higher value in such a material possession, since it only serves our own needs and thus cannot be above us.

On the other hand, if we truly seek money for the benefit of others, then it is not the money itself that we are honoring but the people that we are trying to aid. Seeking money in this case provides a vehicle that allows us to help others, which then promotes our sense of purpose or spirituality.

Prayer is one of the most powerful vehicles that heightens our spirituality. This is why religion and spirituality are often used synonymously. It is because those that pray to God often become more spiritual through the process. In essence, they worship a power that is beyond their own self and from this worship they attain enlightenment.

Of course, not everyone who prays or participates in spiritual rituals is spiritual. Take for example, certain cults or groups that perform acts or deeds for personal gratification or pleasure. Worse yet, there are some who call themselves religious but act in a way that hurts others. These are clearly not spiritual people. A truly spiritual person has a sense of purpose or mission not for pleasure or harm, but to serve mankind.

At the core of any spiritual belief system, including every major religion, we must all adhere to one basic constant in our quest for spirituality. This basic principle is that we worship God or a higher power by protecting and helping others.

Unfortunately, there will always be some people who are susceptible to social or political propaganda and neglect this spiritual constant. This neglect has led to many wars and created unnecessary suffering for millions of people around the world. For the majority of people however, true spirituality can be achieved through their chosen faith by practicing acts of kindness and thoughts of good intention for all human beings.

Practicing the inner work of spirituality is usually described as prayer or meditation. The traditional definition of prayer is communication with a higher power or God. Most religions practice this either alone or in community and both silently and verbally. In this respect, we are communicating our petitions and praise *to* God.

Meditation, however, requires neither communication nor petition or praise, although it may invoke God. This silencing of the mind creates an environment in which thoughts and anxieties cannot penetrate. It is an environment which welcomes God into our minds and hearts, thus creating both peace and calm.

Those who practice prayer and meditation do so with the idea of praising God but also to obtain spirituality through understanding and enlightenment. The spiritual depths that we reach in prayer or meditation helps to clarify our purpose, and therefore opens our hearts and minds to serving others.

As I have alluded to already, meditation is also useful for stress reduction by finding clarity of mind. Some other calming techniques that we have previously discussed include visualization, deep or controlled breathing and focused cognitive (thought) change.

VOLUNTEERISM:

So far, we have discussed obtaining spirituality through our family life, our work and through our practice of faith. In all cases, the common thread involves a sense of purpose that is fulfilled by elevating another person or entity above our self.

Another common activity that can benefit our self as well as society is to volunteer. There are numerous ways we can contribute to the betterment of our community. Some involve more of a time commitment than others. However, there are many opportunities that can fit into a busy person's schedule. Almost any skill that you possess or interest that you may have can be used to serve others.

In addition to helping people, another practical benefit of volunteering is that it provides a healthy mental balance in a world that is so often centered on the individual. In essence, it refocuses our concentration on the important things in life, which can be clouded by our daily routines.

Volunteering also allows you to develop new relationships and have a better understanding of people from different walks of life. These experiences often lead to personal satisfaction and the personal growth that comes with gaining a new perspective on the world.

I can openly say that I have learned valuable lessons from each volunteer experience I encountered during my own life and that these activities have helped me become a better person. Although I have accomplished many things that I am proud of in my life – acquiring an Orthopaedic Surgery Diploma from Harvard, obtaining both a Commercial Airplane Pilot Certification and a SCUBA Dive Master Certificate, as well as becoming a published author for a variety of medical journals to name a few – none of these accomplishments compare to the gratification I have received from doing volunteer work.

For example, in January of 2010, I volunteered to help the victims of Haiti after a massive earthquake reduced this nation's capitol city to rubble. In Haiti, my team served many desperate individuals who were seriously injured as a result of the earthquake. Although we encountered deplorable working conditions and significant risks to our personal safety, the ability to help people was both personally gratifying and spiritually uplifting. Through this kind of volunteer work we learn the true meaning of community, realizing that we are all in this world together, we are obligated to one another and our purpose on earth is to serve each other to the best of our abilities.

Of course, volunteering does not have to involve a stressful situation or be overly challenging. I serve on several volunteer committees that deal with improving health care delivery in my community. Sometimes our work involves only modest or small changes, but this too is beneficial because these efforts may impact the lives of those we aim to serve. Although we may not always be able to make sweeping changes, the effort that we put forth to help others is both rewarding and personally gratifying. And this, of course, goes a long way toward developing our spirituality.

Finding a way to volunteer is very easy. Usually, the more difficult part is following through with this conviction. Like all of the other components of healthy living, volunteering requires dedication. Of course, we all have jobs and families to tend to, but giving just a little of our time has tremendous benefits both to our community at large and for our own personal spiritual growth.

I have provided you with a short list of possible opportunities that may exist in your community right now. Please take a look at all of these options to see if one of these choices may be a good fit for you.

Some ways you can become a volunteer right now include:

> ➢ Work at a homeless shelter cooking, serving food or offering administrative support
> ➢ Spend some time over the holidays volunteering for a "toys for tots" program
> ➢ Offer your services in a crisis center or on a crisis hotline
> ➢ Participate in a fund raising event or raise money for your favorite charitable organization
> ➢ Work as a volunteer in a hospital as a patient sitter or liaison
> ➢ Work in an after school program as a big brother or big sister
> ➢ Help coach kids in school sports or club programs
> ➢ Offer your assistance with the elderly at a senior home or retirement community
> ➢ Spend time counseling people at a local health clinic
> ➢ Offer mentorship to someone who may be interested in your line of work
> ➢ Join groups such as Habitat for Humanity that help improve the living situation of others
> ➢ Help out at your local church, temple or place of worship
> ➢ Volunteer at a day care center or help children with special needs
> ➢ Help a neighbor in need of assistance with a little work around their house or offer to deliver their groceries from time to time

There are literally hundreds of ways that you can offer your services right now. For more information regarding volunteer activities or programs, you can look through the want ads of your local newspaper or check online for opportunities in your area. You will learn a great deal about yourself and others from this experience.

BEATING ADDICTION:

Although we addressed several habitual stresses and addictive habits in our section on stress management, a more thorough discussion concerning addiction is highly relevant to our topic on spirituality. Addiction leads to a major detour on our path to discovery and obscures our purpose or meaning in life. As we have said, our minds need clarity and peace. Addiction in any form creates chaos and unrest which inhibits our ability for spiritual growth.

First let's examine the legal drugs, alcohol and tobacco. We know that these have very toxic effects on the body and can do great harm. Furthermore, we also know there is a dose-related effect. In other words, the more we consume, the risk of addiction as well as physical damage becomes greater.

These substances alter our body both physically and mentally. The physical component occurs when the body itself becomes dependent on these chemicals. This leads to withdraw symptoms when trying to quit or reduce the intake of the substance. To say it another way, the lack of alcohol or nicotine from tobacco, for example, can actually cause a physical reaction in the body of those who are addicted that makes it difficult to quit.

For example, people who crave nicotine often become jittery, irritable and anxious. Headaches, stomach aches or other symptoms of illness can occur after they quit. Alcohol withdraw can be even more severe. People undergoing alcohol withdraw can experience rapid changes in blood pressure or heart rate, dizziness, confusion, delirium, seizures and even death if the physical dependence is severe. For these reasons alone, it is extremely difficult for people who abuse tobacco and alcohol to quit.

What about the mental component of addiction? This can be just as powerful and last much longer than the actual physical component. It is the mental part of the addiction which explains why people often slip or fall back into a pattern of abuse despite having successfully quit for months or even years. The chemicals in these substances create a sense of temporary euphoria or pleasure that is remembered and stored in certain areas of our brain. Over time, our brain chemistry can change and our mind can become dependent on this sense of temporary pleasure or vice. Even though the chemical itself is long gone, the effect of the chemical on our brain remains.

In a manner of speaking, addiction is the antithesis of spirituality because spirituality allows us the freedom to transcend our mind and improve our state of well-being. Addiction, on the other hand, transforms our mind. It enslaves us by creating the need for constant gratification, leading to a viscous self-perpetuating spiral that damages our health and well-being.

There are many examples of addiction, and all have a negative effect on the mind and therefore a negative effect on our overall health. Similar to alcohol and tobacco, sleeping pills, pain killers and illegal drugs are serious addictions that can lead even to death. Some people may be addicted to gambling. Others may have an addiction to food. Addiction to pornography or sex is yet another example.

Addiction occurs when a dependent or abusive behavior causes either harm to our health or negatively affects our personal, work or social life. Although spirituality helps in the treatment of addiction, it is perhaps most useful as a deterrent. To combat addiction, we must seek refuge in spirituality. In other words, we must find our sense of purpose to help free ourselves from the slavery of addiction. As the saying goes "an ounce of prevention is worth a pound of cure."

THOUGHTS AND EMOTIONS:

Emotions play an important role in finding deeper meaning and purpose in life. We have previously discussed how our thoughts can have positive or negative effects on our health. For example, we know that we can reduce stress and anxiety by choosing to have a positive outlook and learning to use a positive internal monologue. In a very similar manner, positive emotions are conducive to spirituality, while negative emotions interfere with our ability to find purpose and meaning. Let's examine a common uplifting emotion that helps transform the spirit....

Love, is an emotion that creates a state of relaxation and peace. Furthermore, true love itself may be a form of spirituality, since it often involves holding another in higher esteem than one's own self. Anger, on the other hand is a negative emotion that makes it difficult for the mind to find purpose or meaning. It creates conflict and disarray and therefore should be avoided as much as possible in one's pursuit of health and wellness.

Some common negative and positive emotions are as follows:

POSITIVE EMOTIONS	NEGATIVE EMOTIONS
LOVE	HATE
JOY	ANGER
HAPPINESS	SADNESS
SURPRISE	FEAR

We must acknowledge that we all feel a wide range of emotions and thoughts. It is unrealistic to believe that we can control our mind to such a degree that all feelings become positive. The most important message is that our thoughts and emotions have a cumulative effect on our well-being. The more often we allow these negative emotions to persist, the more lost and confused we become, which decreases our sense of purpose and our health.

On the other side, the more frequently we allow positive emotions to enter our mind, the more at peace we become, which facilitates our spirituality and improves our health. Thus, our mind must continually balance various thoughts and emotions which ultimately have a significant effect on our overall well-being.

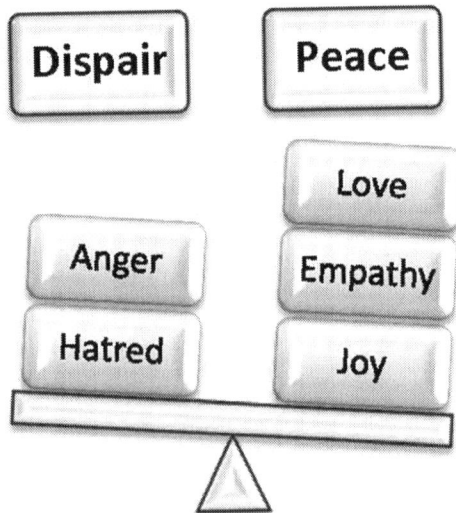

It behooves all of us to frequently exercise our minds in order to maximize positive feelings and minimize the negative ones. A critical first step in training our brain to accept positive thoughts and avoid negative ones is early recognition of a detrimental thought or emotion. Without early detection, these thoughts may continue unchecked leading to escalating anger, hostility and stress which ultimately can lead to physical and/or mental illnesses.

Although most of us know that a certain thought may be negative, it is important to spend time thinking about the common emotions and thoughts that occur throughout our day. For instance, if anger or fear is a common emotion that you feel, ask yourself when specifically does this occur and how does it affect your emotional and physical well-being. Equally important, when experiencing love or joy, ask yourself when is it that you feel this and how does it affect you. This by no means is a trivial exercise, indeed it is a critical first step in the early recognition of our thoughts.

In addition, we must constantly monitor our thoughts and emotions while they are happening to us, especially the negative ones. For example, at the moment a negative emotion such as sadness or anger enters our mind, do not allow this emotion to guide you to feel or act in a certain manner.

Rather, vow to replace this emotion with one that is positive. Remind yourself that these negative thoughts only hurt you in the long run. Even if you feel wronged by another, remember that allowing a negative emotion to run free in your mind only creates more pain and suffering.

Many times we allow negative emotions to gain control of our thoughts as a misguided attempt to obtain closure or obtain peace. Although this is counterproductive to our goal, it happens to all of us frequently and we must constantly strive to change the way we think in order to truly acquire resolution or calm.

Just think about how you feel when you are driving your car and another person cuts you off or does something you believe is inappropriate. The first emotion that often surfaces is anger and a verbal or mental outburst such as "that --------, what the -------- is that person doing!" (insert your own oft-used insults). Some people may even alter the way they are driving in order to show the other person that they are angry. So why do we react this way? What purpose does it serve?

Sometimes we react this way because we feel we were put in danger, and fear or anxiety has taken over during this circumstance. Other times we feel that we were wronged or mistreated by another person. In either case, what we all truly want is peace and closure. We may wrongly believe that directing anger or even acting out towards another person may bring us our needed closure. However, it never does. This is because we are trying to obtain resolution for a negative emotion by using a negative thought.

Anger often leads to hostility or worsening of our negative emotions rather than dampening them. You may recognize this when a seemingly small event leads you to fixate on your thoughts and you find yourself reliving the troubling event throughout the day. Actually, we should be seeking closure through positive thinking. For example, in the circumstance where we may have felt endangered in our vehicle, the first step after the event has occurred is to recognize the negative emotion. Say to yourself, I am feeling angry or I feel scared.

Next, remind yourself that negative emotions are a misguided attempt at obtaining closure. Understand that continuing these negative thoughts will never bring you closure. It has the opposite effect of leading you farther away from conflict resolution.

Use the process of positive thought reinforcement to resolve these negative thoughts or emotions. It helps to come up with several common phrases or sentences to assist you in finding peace whenever a troubling event has caused you to become angered or upset. You can repeat the following phrases to yourself:

"Everything is okay now"

"I am safe"

"No harm has been done"

"We all make mistakes and I forgive"

"Getting angry or mad only hurts me and I won't allow that to happen to me"

"I've also caused others to become angry or sad in the past"

The actual phrase that you choose is up to you so long as it reinforces true closure. The defining element that all of these positive thoughts have in common are empathy or forgiveness. Striving for forgiveness does not mean that we are weak or cowardly people. On the contrary, it takes enormous strength to forgive others, including ourselves, and it ultimately allows us to find peace, tranquility and happiness.

DIET, EXERCISE AND STRESS REDUCTION:

Lastly, an obvious and commonly referring theme of the Healthy 4 program is the interwoven relationship that exists between our four health components. We know that proper diet, exercise, stress reduction and spirituality combine to optimize our health and well-being and that practicing each individual component strengthens the next. Therefore, living healthier is another common path towards spirituality. In other words, proper diet, exercise and stress reduction are also methods that promote spirituality. Thus, you began preparing your mind for heightened spirituality from the beginning of this book.

Reflect for a moment on our stress management techniques. We know that these reduce anxiety and promote calm which leads to an improved clarity of mind. As your mind relaxes, your ability to find deeper meaning in life improves tremendously. This is why many people who practice meditation or prayer strongly believe that it leads to a path of enlightenment.

Let's look at two other examples related to diet and exercise. At some point or another we have all consumed a large, unhealthy meal or remained sedentary in our home for an entire day watching television or doing nothing. During these periods an interesting phenomenon occurs. We usually feel fatigue and lethargic.

On the other side, we know that eating a healthy meal and performing some exercise leaves us feeling more invigorated and focused. This energy and focus are important prerequisites that allow us to positively transform our mind and improve our spirituality.

Similar to diet, exercise and stress reduction, spirituality is never an absolute. Rather it exists as a continuum with infinite possibilities. Spirituality, like the other health components, is dynamic and requires attention throughout our life.

Before approaching the final chapter and conclusion of our Healthy 4 program, let's review some methods that we have at our disposal to find our sense of purpose and heighten our spirituality. Transforming the mind through these or any other techniques never occurs quickly or without effort. It takes dedication and a willingness to change.

PRACTICES THAT PROMOTE SPIRITUALITY:

- ➢ Find meaning in your work by focusing on helping others
- ➢ Avoid searching for happiness from financial or material gain
- ➢ Spend quality time with family and nurture these relationships
- ➢ Build meaningful friendships
- ➢ Clear your mind and create peace through meditation, deep breathing or visualization techniques
- ➢ Manage stress
- ➢ Eat a healthy diet
- ➢ Exercise
- ➢ Practice your faith or religion
- ➢ Volunteer or spend some time helping others in need
- ➢ Seek help for your addictions
- ➢ Focus on the strengths of others rather than their weaknesses
- ➢ Remind yourself that "forgiveness is divine"
- ➢ Tell someone that you love them
- ➢ Avoid excessive alcohol or tobacco use
- ➢ Smile, greet or be kind to a stranger that passes you by
- ➢ Discourage negative emotions
- ➢ Nurture positive emotions
- ➢ Think about helping others before yourself

CHAPTER FIFTEEN:
PUTTING IT ALL TOGETHER

In our final chapter we begin by reviewing how spirituality benefits, not just our mental health, but our physical health as well. We then combine the key concepts and techniques that you have learned from each of the health components into a single program. This Healthy 4 program is your guide to optimal health and should be used as a reference whenever necessary.

All of us are familiar with the proverb "the more we give, the more we shall receive." From a practical point of view, this is exactly what spirituality offers to us because practicing spirituality will elevate our mind and improve our health. Let's examine some of the physical effects that spirituality has on the body.

Everyone one of us knows that helping others tends to improve our own mood and brings us significant joy. Moreover, the peace and joy that we receive by serving either a higher power or a fellow human being tends to be enduring. In other words, the benefits that we receive by satisfying our spiritual side greatly outlast the temporary pleasures that we may feel when satisfying our own self interests.

For example, enjoying an excellent meal or drinking a nice glass of wine may be very gratifying in the moment, but once we are finished it does nothing else for us. Although we may remember it for awhile, it does not continue to bring us pleasure once the actual event is over.

On the other hand, the joy that you bring others by volunteering just a few hours of your time to help deliver food to needy families during the holidays may stay with you forever. This self sacrificing memory, in contrast to the previous self serving memory, will continue to bring you joy and focus your mind on positive thoughts for a very long time.

With each positive thought and emotion our mind evolves and becomes more positive as a result. On the other hand, negative feelings tend to reinforce future negative thoughts. Science is only just beginning to understand how our thoughts affect our brain chemistry. All indications point to the fact that positive thinking does play an important role in our mental and physical health.

As we have alluded to earlier, constant worry and anxiety can lead to increased stress on our body. This stress has been associated with many diseases including depression and other mental illnesses, heart disease, ulcers, digestive tract syndromes, increased susceptibility to infectious diseases and cancer. On the other hand, feeling a sense of calm and happiness can combat all these problems and help to fight off disease.

Reflect on your own life for a minute and recall times of significant personal stress or unhappiness. During these times, many of you may recall having trouble sleeping, fatigue, stomach aches, nausea, heartburn, diarrhea or constipation, headaches, muscle aches, an irregular heart beat or a common cold. This list of symptoms sounds like the side effects of a bad drug. In fact, that's just what stress and negative emotions are.

Think about drugs like alcohol and nicotine, these are external toxins that damage your body with cumulative exposure. In a similar manner, the excessive hormones and chemicals that the body produces with negative thinking and stress are essentially toxic internal drugs that can damage your physical body. This is why both stress reduction and spirituality are so vital to any health program and why we integrate all four health components into one program.

FINAL THOUGHTS:

Before we review the final summary plan, let me add just a few last words about the Healthy 4 program. It is expected that making spiritual progress will appear to take longer than our other areas of health. However, this does not make it any less significant. In fact, the first three components of diet, exercise and stress reduction help to prepare one's mind in the quest for higher purpose or spirituality. Thus, the suggested methodologies to enhance your spiritual side are listed in the last stage of the program designated as "Beyond 90 days."

Obviously, this does not mean that you will avoid activities that might promote spirituality early in the plan. However, the emphasis on this last component of health has been placed at the end of the program for good reason. This is to avoid early overload and to allow you to progressively focus on the important initial stages of diet, exercise and stress management. Once these routines are established, it becomes easier to put it all together in order to optimize your health and ensure enduring results.

At first glance, this program may appear to be a significant amount of work. Now that we have discussed all of these concepts and techniques in each of the previous sections, we can see that most of these tips are efficient and easy to follow when applied in steps. The duration of each stage in this plan has been established to provide you with a platform from which you can continue to build in the future. The true power of the Healthy 4 system does not come from this platform itself. Rather, it comes from integrating the techniques from each of the four components to the best of your abilities and continuing them throughout your lifetime.

This program is your guide to greater health and vitality. To return to our earlier automobile analogy, the outline that I have provided is the road map (GPS for all you techies) and you are the vehicle. Just like the car with four wheels, this program targets the principle four components of health. Neglecting one or more of these components is equivalent to driving on one or more flat tires. You can still operate your vehicle, but it is much less efficient and eventually it will lead to a breakdown. In order for your body to run smoothly, you must integrate all four components into your life and ensure that they are properly balanced.

Your reading throughout this book has provided you with a solid foundation. Now that you have acquired the necessary knowledge and understanding, you are ready to use this outline. If you would like to print a similar copy of this program summary on line, you can download it at www.Healthy4.com. Remember to refer to the specific chapters in the book whenever you need to refresh your memory or find inspiration.

Believe in this program and believe in yourself and the rewards will be substantial! I wish each and every one of you success and prosperity, and I thank you for the privilege of allowing me to help optimize your health. It's now time to review the key to unlocking greater health and well-being...

Healthy 4

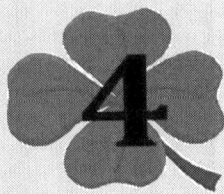

THE COMPLETE HEALTHY 4 PROGRAM:

DAY 1 – DAY 15:

❖ Diet: Begin recording your daily calorie consumption each day for the first 15 days (review nutrition labels and continue your normal dietary habits)

❖ Exercise Program: None (continue normal activity and exercise routines)

❖ Stress Management Tips and Techniques:
  ✓ Utilize visualization methods
  ✓ Controlled breathing techniques
  ✓ Try meditation
  ✓ Use postural techniques: tai chi, yoga or routine stretching
  ✓ Access your social network and talk with others
  ✓ Start a new hobby
  ✓ Use biofeedback
  ✓ Ensure adequate sleep hygiene
  ✓ Reduce caffeine and alcohol intake
  ✓ Avoid tobacco
  ✓ Exercise
  ✓ Maintain a proper diet
  ✓ Avoid the stressor if appropriate
  ✓ Focus on positive thoughts/develop a healthy internal monologue

<u>DAY 16 – DAY 30:</u>

❖ Diet: Continue recording your daily calorie consumption
❖ Diet: Use the information from your calorie consumption log to establish a daily calorie consumption limit (example: 2000 calories/day)
❖ Diet: Use the following dieting pearls to assist you:
   ✓ Avoid eating until full
   ✓ Eat small portions or reduce your meal size
   ✓ Eat <u>more</u> frequently during the day versus one or two large meals
   ✓ Don't wait until your hunger is strong before you eat
   ✓ SLOW DOWN when you eat
   ✓ Pack your own food and carry nutritional supplements with you
   ✓ Avoid eating as a reflex to hunger (assess for abnormal cues)
   ✓ Avoid buffets and all you can eat menus
   ✓ Consume low calorie foods and drinks
   ✓ Count your calories and set daily goals
   ✓ Keep yourself well hydrated
   ✓ Drink water rather high calorie drinks
   ✓ Try a healthy snack <u>before</u> a meal
   ✓ Forget about adhering to traditional course meals (i.e. 3 or 4 courses)
   ✓ DON'T feel the need to clear your plate and STOP eating once you meet your dietary goals
   ✓ Never eat before going to sleep
   ✓ Associate positive thought to healthy foods
   ✓ Eat a well-balanced diet
   ✓ Consume most of your fats from **un**saturated, **non**-trans fat sources
   ✓ Don't prepare or cover your food with unhealthy toppings

❖ Exercise Program: Start beginner exercise program (or higher level depending on comfort and previous experience)

<u>Level One – Beginner:</u>

<u>Day 1 Exercise Program (Day 16 Overall Wellness Program):</u>
    Cardio training: 30 minutes elliptical machine, swimming, stationary bike or equivalent
    Core resistance training: push ups and/or bench press 2 sets
    Core resistance training: pull ups and/or pull downs 2 sets
    Sit ups: 2 sets

<u>Day 2: Rest</u>

<u>Day 3:</u>
    Cardio training: 30 minutes elliptical machine, swimming, stationary bike or equivalent
    Core resistance training: squats 2 sets
    Sit ups: 2 sets

<u>Day 4: Rest</u>

<u>Day 5:</u>
    Cardio training: 30 minutes elliptical machine, swimming, stationary bike or equivalent
    Core resistance training: push ups and/or bench press 2 sets
    Core resistance training: pull ups and/or pull downs 2 sets
    Sit ups: 2 sets

<u>Day 6 & 7: Rest then Repeat</u>

❖ Stress Management: Continue using tips and techniques

DAY 31 – 90:

❖ Diet: Refine calorie consumption goals every one to two weeks as needed

❖ Diet: Continue using daily calorie consumption log book

❖ Exercise: Continue exercise program and advance level when comfortable

Level Two – Intermediate Exercise Program:

Day 1:
  Cardio training: 30 minutes elliptical machine, swimming, stationary bike or equivalent
  Core resistance training: push ups and/or bench press 3 sets
  Core resistance training: pull ups and/or pull downs 3 sets
  Sit ups: 2-3 sets

Day 2: Rest

Day 3:
  Cardio training: 30 minutes elliptical machine, swimming, stationary bike or equivalent
  Core resistance training: squats 2-3 sets
  Sit ups: 2-3 sets

Day 4: Rest

Day 5:
  Cardio training: 30 minutes elliptical machine, swimming, stationary bike or equivalent
  Core resistance training: push ups and/or bench press 3 sets
  Core resistance training: pull ups and/or pull downs 3 sets
  Sit ups: 2-3 sets

Day 6: Rest

Day 7: Rest or Repeat

Or Alternatively:

Level Three – Advanced Exercise Program:

Day 1:
    Cardio training: 30 minutes elliptical machine, swimming, stationary bike or equivalent
    Core resistance training: push ups and/or bench press: 4 sets
    Core resistance training: pull ups and/or pull downs: 4 sets

Day 2:
    Cardio training: 30 minutes elliptical machine, swimming, stationary bike or equivalent
    Core resistance training: squats: 3 sets
    Sit ups: 3 sets

Day 3: Rest

Day 4:
    Cardio training: 30 minutes elliptical machine, swimming, stationary bike or equivalent
    Core resistance training: push ups and/or bench press: 4 sets
    Core resistance training: pull ups and/or pull downs: 4 sets

Day 5:
    Cardio training: 30 minutes elliptical machine, swimming, stationary bike or equivalent
    Core resistance training: squats: 3 sets
    Sit ups: 3 sets

Day 6: Rest

Day 7: Rest or Repeat

❖ Stress Management: Continue using tips and techniques

Beyond Day 90:

❖ Diet: Continue lifelong learning and perfecting

❖ Exercise: Continue lifelong learning and perfecting

❖ Stress Management: Continue lifelong learning and perfecting

❖ Spirituality Tips and Techniques:
  ✓ Find meaning in your work by focusing on helping others
  ✓ Avoid searching for happiness from financial or material gain
  ✓ Spend quality time with family
  ✓ Nurture relationships thru open communication and em-pathy
  ✓ Build meaningful friendships with others
  ✓ Focus your mind using meditation
  ✓ Use controlled breathing to improve your state of relaxa-tion
  ✓ Use visualization to create a sense of calm
  ✓ Manage your stress
  ✓ Eat a healthy diet
  ✓ Maintain good sleep habits
  ✓ Exercise
  ✓ Practice your faith or religion regularly
  ✓ Volunteer or spend some time helping others in need
  ✓ Seek help for your addictions
  ✓ Focus on the strengths of others rather than their weak-nesses

✓ Remind yourself that "forgiveness is divine"
✓ Tell someone that you love them
✓ Avoid excessive alcohol or tobacco use
✓ Smile, greet or be kind to a stranger that passes you by
✓ Discourage negative emotions
✓ Nurture positive emotions
✓ Think about helping others before yourself
✓ Begin lifelong learning and perfecting these techniques....

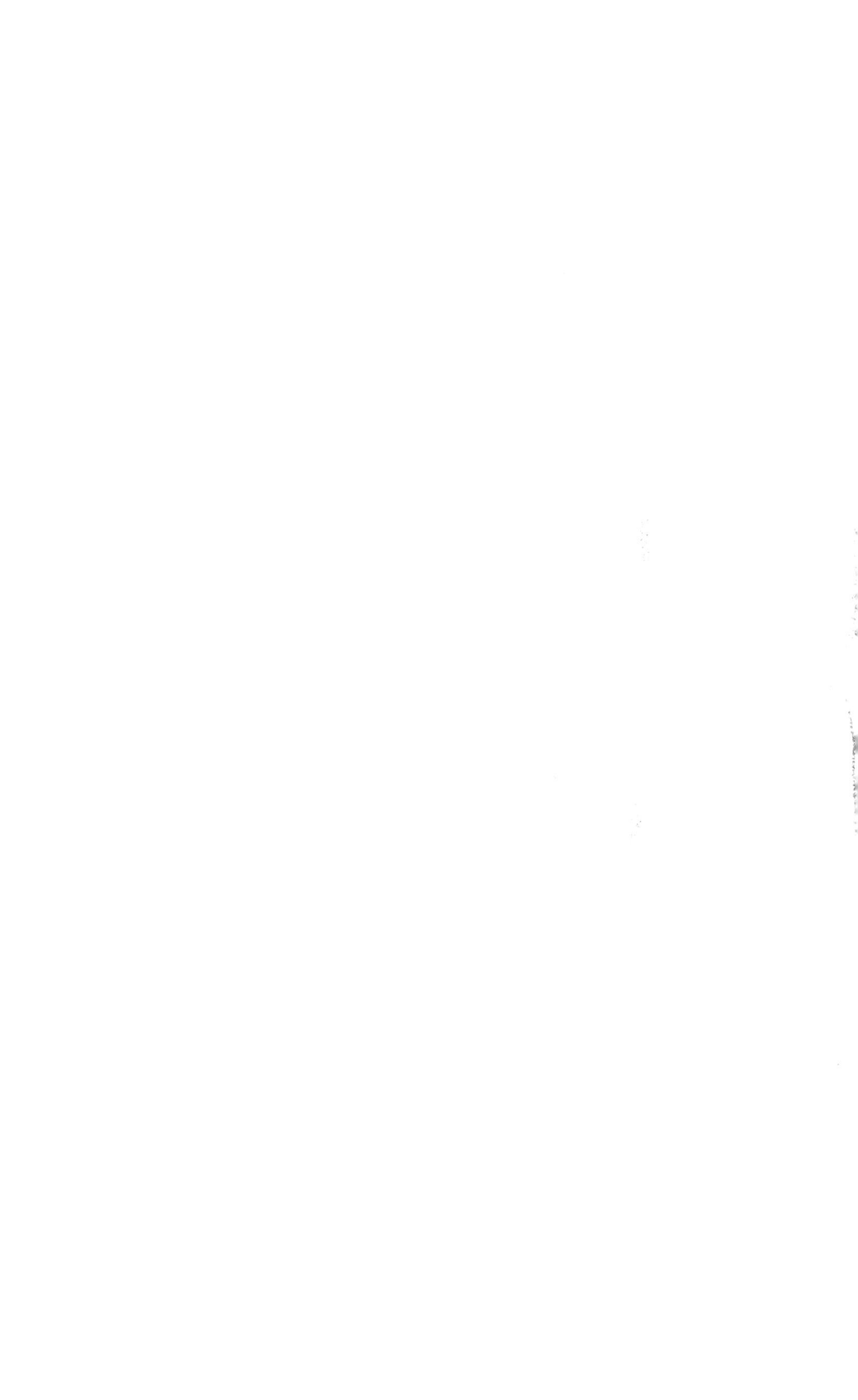